International Perspectives on Sport and Exercise Psychology

Psychology of Sport Excellence

International Perspectives on Sport and Exercise Psychology

Psychology of Sport Excellence

TSUNG-MIN HUNG

RONNIE LIDOR

DIETER HACKFORT

EDITORS

Dieter Hackfort and Gershon Tenenbaum
Series Editors-in-Chief

Fitness Information Technology
A Division of the International Center for Performance Excellence
262 Coliseum, WVU-PASS • P O Box 6116 • Morgantown, WV 26506-6116

Library of Congress Card Catalog Number: 2008940701

ISBN: 978-1-885693-90-7

Production Editor: Matt Brann
Cover Design: 40 West Studios
Typesetter: 40 West Studios
Copyeditor: Danielle Costello
Proofreader: Maria E. denBoer
Indexer: Maria E. denBoer
Printed by: Sheridan Books

10 9 8 7 6 5 4 3 2 1

Fitness Information Technology
A Division of the International Center for Performance Excellence
West Virginia University
262 Coliseum, WVU-PASS
PO Box 6116
Morgantown, WV 26506-6116
800.477.4348 (toll free)
304.293.6888 (phone)
304.293.6658 (fax)
Email: fitcustomerservice@mail.wvu.edu
Website: www.fitinfotech.com

Table of Contents

Table of Contents

FOREWORD

This new series, titled *International Perspectives on Sport and Exercise Psychology*, aims at providing a sequence of topics organized by outstanding and internationally respected experts in their fields. The advantage of editing a collection of articles within one volume lies in its freedom from the space constraints typical of journal articles (even special issues are limited in space) such as the ones published in the *International Journal of Sport and Exercise Psychology* (IJSEP) and other journals in the field. The volumes that are planned to be included in this series center on essential issues in the field, and represent the most up-to-date information on these subjects. This series is open to a broad scope of topics that represent various theoretical perspectives and methodological approaches, and provides a cross-cultural exchange of ideas and insights. It is our hope that international discussion targeted toward global understanding will follow.

The first book in the series is entitled *Psychology of Sport Excellence*. The contributions to this volume consist of presentations made by members of the Managing Council (MC) of the International Society of Sport Psychology (ISSP) on the occasion of an international symposium held in Taipei, Taiwan, in 2006.

The chapters were compiled and reviewed by the editors of this volume, Tsung-Min Hung, ISSP MC member, Ronnie Lidor, general secretary of the ISSP, and Dieter Hackfort, president of the ISSP. The chapters present the research and perspectives of colleagues from five continents. We hope that the readers will find this first volume especially interesting, as it consists of the views of scientists and researchers representing some countries and cultures not typically published in the English language.

Based on more than a decade of cooperation and collaboration within the ISSP, and as the founding co-editors of the *IJSEP*, we believe that the *International Perspectives on Sport and Exercise Psychology* series will offer a platform for the exchange of scientific information that will complement the journal and the special issues of the journal, by providing extended and diversified elaboration on topics of fundamental interest and importance to those working in the field.

We are very pleased to collaborate again with Fitness Information Technology (FIT), which is serving as the publisher of this series. The publication of this series, as well as the publication of the *IJSEP*—the official journal of the ISSP—makes FIT the "home publisher" of the ISSP, and, thus, the leading publisher of sport and exercise psychology worldwide.

Dieter Hackfort and Gershon Tenenbaum
Series Editors-in-Chief

ACKNOWLEDGMENTS

The editors would like to express their deepest appreciation to all the individuals who contributed chapters to this book; their cooperation and enthusiasm were key factors in its completion. We would like to thank the members of the International Society of Sport Psychology (ISSP) Managing Council (2005-2009) for their support and guidance throughout the preparation of this book. In addition, we would like to acknowledge the work done by Dinah Olswang from the Zinman College of Physical Education and Sport Sciences at the Wingate Institute (Israel). Her assistance in preparing each chapter was instrumental in our goal of achieving uniformity throughout the book. Finally, we extend our appreciation to editor Matthew Brann and the rest of the staff at Fitness Information Technology, a division of the International Center for Performance Excellence at West Virginia University (USA), for their support and encouragement during each phase of the preparation of this book.

CHAPTER 1

Achieving Excellence in Sport— The Psychological Edge

RONNIE LIDOR, DIETER HACKFORT, AND TSUNG-MIN HUNG

Introduction

Achieving excellence in sport, as well as in other domains such as art, music, and science, is a multifaceted journey that requires the right combination of human talent and task-pertinent environmental support (Bloom, 1985; Howe, 1999). This journey to the top level of human performance may last a number of years, during which the individual must focus on skill improvement in a well-developed, supervised training program (see Côté, Lidor, & Hackfort, in press). In essence, this training program should provide the individual with instructional conditions that will encourage motivation and enable improvement and refinement of the skills required for high-level achievement.

Individuals who set an exceptional goal for themselves eagerly strive to formulate a clear plan of how to achieve this goal. This formula should be comprised of factors that are considered to be key contributors to achieving excellence in a particular domain. Among the potential factors are those associated with the talent level of the individual or with his or her inherent traits (i.e., nature's edge), as well as those that reflect the contribution of environmental components involved in the development of the individual, such as the knowledge and experience of his or her mentors, or the amount of time and practice one is willing to invest in the specific domain (i.e., nurture's edge).

While it is easy to apply components that have the greatest potential to contribute to the individual's goal, it is much harder to assess, in a precise manner, the exact weight each component lends to success. For example, one individual who reaches the pinnacle of success in a given domain might have adequate but not extraordinary talent. However, this individual regularly worked hard with leading mentors who helped to substantially improve his or her abilities, and thus he or she was able to achieve excellence despite a relatively low level of talent. In another case, a very talented individual reaches a high level of proficiency although he or she did not have the opportunity to receive help from the professional community, and therefore the journey to the top level relied mainly on the individual's natural talent and willpower. Consequently, it can be postulated that there are various pathways of achievement that can be observed and followed.

A similar observation can be made for those individuals who reached the summit in the domain of sport—there are different ways to reach the top. Various retrospective studies (e.g., Hemery, 1986; Kalinowski, 1985a, b; Monsaas, 1985) review articles and chapters (e.g., Hackfort, 2006; Johnson & Tenenbaum, 2006; Singer & Janelle, 1999), and conference proceedings (e.g., Schilling & Herren, 1985) have indicated that athletes can attain excellence through various pathways that utilize different combinations of those components found to be contributors to success in sport (e.g., physical attributes, psychological traits, and environmental support). Some elite athletes reported that they achieved their proficiency mainly because of good physical attributes (e.g., endurance, agility, speed, and strength), which enabled them to gain a clear advantage over their counterparts (Fisher & Borms, 1990; Hemery, 1986). Others stressed the importance of the support they received from their coaches in different phases of their athletic career, particularly at the early phases of talent development (Kalinowski, 1985a, b). Another group of athletes attributed their success to the sport consultants who worked with them and helped them deal with psychological issues related to their sports, such as coping with injuries, focusing attention, and coping with failure (Hemery, 1986; Orlick, 2000; Vernacchia, McGuire, & Cook, 1992).

Regardless of the precise contribution of components derived from both nature and nurture—or any combination of these components—it is obvious that the quality of the professional support with which the elite athlete is provided throughout his or her career is a key factor in the long journey to achieving peak performance (Johnson & Tenenbaum, 2006; Lidor, Côté, & Hackfort, in press; Singer & Janelle, 1999). In elite individual and team sports, typical professional support aims at working with the elite athlete in four different preparations: physical, technical, tactical, and psychological (Bompa, 1999; Lidor, Blumenstein, & Tenenbaum, 2007). In effective professional support, interrelationships should exist among all four preparations if the elite athlete expects to receive the greatest benefit from the entire preparation program. In this book, *Psychology of Sport Excellence,* contributions are presented to examine and explain the impact of one of these preparations on elite athletes in their journey to attain excellence—the psychological preparation. The chapters included in this book discuss various theoretical and practical issues related to the use of psychological programs in elite individual and team sports.

The Development and Objectives of the Book

The idea of developing this book emerged during an international seminar entitled *The International Forum of the Psychology of Olympic Excellence* held in Taiwan in October, 2006. The seminar was organized in a combined effort of the *International Society of Sport Psychology* (ISSP) and *The Society for Sport and Exercise Psychology of Taiwan.* Our intention was to include as chapters in the book the contributions from the keynote speakers who had been invited to the seminar to share their scientific and applied experience. Each invited speaker was asked to submit a paper on his or her topic at the time of the seminar. All speakers agreed to do so, some of them collaborating with other authors in preparing their chapters. Each chapter included in this volume was subsequently extended and updated for publication by the authors after the seminar.

The objective of this volume is threefold. First, to examine theoretical and practical aspects of the use of psychological preparation in elite sports; second, to present the psychological interventions, strategies, and techniques utilized by sport psychology consultants who have worked with elite athletes for many years; third, to describe the philosophies of consultation, procedures to be used, and consultation frameworks of sport psychology consultants working with elite athletes representing different cultures in different regions and continents around the globe, such as Africa, Asia, Europe, and North America.

An attempt was made in this book to integrate theoretical knowledge emerging from empirical inquiries in sport psychology with applied knowledge gained by sport psychology consultants who had worked with athletes in different sports, based on their long years of experience. This knowledge can be used in psychological preparations aimed at helping elite athletes in individual and team sports improve their psychological skills and mental readiness for the practice, game, or competition.

The Structure of the Book

This book consists of thirteen chapters. Chapter 1, "Achieving Excellence in Sport—The Psychological

Edge" (Ronnie Lidor, Dieter Hackfort, and Tsung-Min Hung), is an introductory chapter that provides the rationale and objectives of the book. In addition, the background of each chapter included in the book (i.e., Chapters 2 to 13) is provided.

Chapter 2, "The Action Theory-Based Mental Test and Training System (MTTS)" (Dieter Hackfort, Conor Kilgallen, and Liu Hao), reports on the development of a Mental Test and Training System (MTTS), which integrates computer-assisted tools and field setups for the testing and training of mental processes and skills deemed important in elite sports. The MTTS, based on the action-theory concept, includes a computerized mental test system, action checks, and a mental training system. The fundamental idea is to create specific person-task-environment constellations as action situations for testing and training purposes. In this chapter, special emphasis is given to performance-oriented tasks, such as kicking a ball and racing tasks.

Chapter 3, "A Sport Psychology Service Delivery Model for Developing and Current Track and Field Athletes and Coaches" (Traci Statler and Keith Henschen), introduces and describes a model of sport psychology service delivery available to track and field athletes in the United States. The first part of the chapter introduces sport psychology practitioners, coaches, and athletes to the short-term, intensive education program presented each summer to some of America's best developing youth track and field athletes. The objective of this program is to share a popular and effective sport psychology consultation model with those seeking an understanding of psychological talent development for potential Olympians. The second part of the chapter describes the ways in which this developmental foundation is further fostered and built upon as the athlete continues to progress and eventually emerges at the elite rank of "Olympian" or "World Champion." The authors explain the guiding purpose and general educational mission of the USA Track & Field (USATF) sport psychology program, which has been an integral part of the development of American track and field athletes since the program's inception in 1982.

Chapter 4, "Olympic Games and Sport Psychology" (Sidónio Serpa), focuses on the psychological preparation given to elite athletes participating in major sport events such as the Olympic Games. The author goes back to the roots of the modern Olympics and claims that Pierre de Coubertin's interest in sport psychology was expressed many times in articles that he wrote from the very beginning of the 20th century. According to Coubertin, the organization of the 1913 *International Congress of Psychology and Physiology of Sports* in Lausanne, Switzerland, aimed at christening a new science, or more precisely, a new branch of science. Coubertin believed that the psychological factors of sport performance should be developed in order to contribute to the athlete's personal growth. Indeed, the development of sport psychology is profoundly associated with the Olympic movement and its founder. The Olympic Games became a major worldwide competition that has significant personal meaning for those who succeeded in participating and achieving their goals in such a unique context. This chapter focuses on the specific constraints that differentiate the Olympic competition from other major sporting events. Thus, special adaptation is required, and psychological strategies and skills should be taught and practiced during the preparation and on-site phases. After the event, debriefing sessions should help athletes make a bridge from this intensive experience to future projects.

Chapter 5, "Sport Psychology Service Provision at Elite International Competition" (Judy L. Van Raalte and Albert J. Petitpas), provides guidelines for sport psychologists traveling and working with elite competitive athletes and teams. There are a number of important issues that applied sport psychologists should consider when planning to provide services at elite international competitions. These include development of an appropriate theoretical approach to service delivery, pre-event preparation, intervention implementation, and program evaluation. In this chapter, each of these key areas is discussed in detail.

Chapter 6, "Free-Throw Shots in Basketball: Physical and Psychological Routines" (Ronnie Lidor), examines the use of preparatory routines by elite basketball players performing free throws during the game. In this chapter an attempt was made to search for the most crucial components that should comprise a successful preparatory routine for free-throw shots in basketball. More specifically, the purpose of this chapter is twofold: (a) to review the literature examining the use of preparatory routines by basketball players when they are preparing themselves for the free-throw shooting act, including physical and psychological routines from the perspective of both research findings and anecdotal evidence, and (b) to suggest a routine that can be used by beginning free-throw shooters or those who have not already established a routine. The chapter also provides a number of practical recommendations for sport psychology consultants who work with beginning and advanced basketball players.

Chapter 7, "Talent Development in Sport: The Perspective of Career Transitions" (Natalia Stambulova), describes three related but different meanings of the term *talent* in sport, emphasizing the biological, psychological, and social perspectives of this phenomenon. The chapter examines the link between talent and career development in sport, where athletic career development, with its normative stages and transitions, serves as a broader context for talent development. Based on the author's multi-year study of career transitions of Russian athletes, perceived career demands and coping resources during six normative athletic transitions are defined, followed by an athletic career transition model that explains the process of transition. In addition, three potential problems that occur when dealing with young prospects, conventionally labeled as "quick progress," "early social recognition," and "one-sided development," are considered from the career-transition perspective. Suggestions for preventing and coping with these problems are provided, emphasizing the importance of collaborative efforts of sport managers, coaches, the athlete's parents, and sport psychologists in approaching young athletes from a holistic lifespan perspective and helping them achieve success, both in sport and in life.

Chapter 8, "Interdisciplinary Teaching, Goal Orientation, Self-Determination, and Responsibility in Life" (Athanasios G. Papaioannou and Dimotrios Milosis), presents selected findings from one study which examined the benefits of the physical education curriculum to junior high school students. This program is based on the multidimensional model of goal orientation and adopted a holistic approach to the teaching process. It was found that some coaches are committed not only to teaching their athletes how to excel in sport, but in life as well. However, while the subject of performance enhancement strategies is a hot topic in sport psychology research, strategies aimed at enhancing personal development and life skills have been studied less often. The physical education program presented in this chapter emphasizes the holistic growth of the individual, including physical, cognitive, emotional, and social development. It is emphasized that the adoption of this theoretical and practical framework by physical educators and coaches will enable them to provide substantial help to their students and athletes so that they will excel not only in sport, but also in school and life.

Chapter 9, "Research on Arab Sport Excellence" (Abderrahim Baria), deals with a number of issues occupying the attention of researchers and practitioners in Arab countries. A brief overview designed to compare the evolution of Arab sport psychology to that of the Western world is presented. In addition, selected results from one study on the psychological ingredients for success and excellence in Arab sports are presented. The findings of this study clearly indicate that Moroccan elite athletes associate several mental elements with excellence in sport. For these athletes, commitment, confidence, distraction control, and positive images seem to be the major factors that determine their success. The study attempted to convey new information on the field of Arab sport excellence. It provides Arab coaches, athletes, and sport administrators with a portrait of how top Arab athletes perceive the elements that lead to superiority in sport, and how they have climbed the ladder to reach the top.

Chapter 10, "The Road to Continued Sport Participation and Sport Excellence" (Jean Côté), discusses one of the major issues related to children's sport programs—to sample (different activities) or to specialize (in one particular activity)? On the one hand, it was proposed that the most economical way of producing talent in sport is to provide sport programs, from ages 6 to 12, that focus on children's physical needs and preferences, not on a rigid skill-based model. Sport programs that focus on play and children's development have been shown to lead to less dropout, continued participation in sport, and elite performance later in life. On the other hand, children's sport programs that focus on a rigid skill-based model imply an early selection of "talented" children, an increase in resources for a special group of athletes, and training that is not always consistent with the children's motivation to participate in sports. As such, some youth sport programs are designed with the long-term objective of producing elite-level athletes instead of serving the short-term needs of children. The chapter provides support for an elite sport performance through a sampling trajectory by emphasizing the various benefits of each pathway.

Chapter 11, "Application of Mental Training with Elite Athletes" (Rico Schuijers), focuses on the work relationship between the sport psychologist and the elite athlete. An overview of the application of mental training is provided, as well as a thorough description of the procedure that the applied sport psychologist should follow while providing sport psychology consultations to elite athletes. This procedure consists of the first contact, decision about continuation, survey and processing of information, analysis of the information, goal setting, executing the mental training plan, and evaluation. In addition, the chapter outlines a number of consultation issues that play a role in improving the quality of the work relationship between the sport psychologist and the athlete, such as the development of the work relationship over time as well as the mistakes/problems that can occur in the mental training sessions.

Chapter 12, "Regulating Mental States through Electroencephalography and Heart Rate Biofeedback Training" (Tsung-Min Hung, Dong-Yang Fong, Yung-Shun Wang, Po-Yi Lin, and Li-Chuan Lo), discusses prominent advancements in psychophysiology and cognitive neuroscience, which show the close relationship between body and mind. More specifically, the chapter introduces biofeedback and review studies utilizing neurofeedback training and heart rate (HR) biofeedback training to enhance sport performance. Biofeedback training is one of the applications of the close body-mind connection. Although the discussion of biofeedback training is limited to electroencephalography (EEG) and HR in this chapter, the intention is to show the great potential of biofeedback in fostering an understanding of how the mind works and how it can relate to sport performance. In sports, both neurofeedback and HR biofeedback have been used with some success in self-regulation. The chapter examines how sport psychologists can use neurofeedback and HR biofeedback in their attempt to understand the optimal mental states of athletes in order to help them control their mind during sport performance.

Chapter 13, "Integrating the Oriental Martial Arts *Chi* Concept into Psychological Skills Training" (Frank J. H. Lu), introduces the concept of *Chi* for the use of applied sport psychologists. *Chi* is an oriental martial arts concept, which, by its simplest definition, represents one's life vital force. However, there is more than vital force in the martial artist's conceptualization of *Chi* when it is used as a tool to promote health or enhance power, or even to control anxiety while performing. Because the practice of *Chi* is similar to the practice of psychological skill training (PST), this concept can naturally be integrated into the psychological prepara-

tion developed for elite athletes. The chapter addresses the link between *Chi* and PST, and presents a number of unique examples that athletes can use while performing in athletic settings. In addition, the concept of *Chi* is connected to achieving Olympic excellence.

In *Psychology of Sport Excellence*, we attempted to present not only research findings that have emerged from empirical inquiries in sport and exercise psychology, but also some perspectives of sport psychology consultants who have been working with elite athletes over a long period of time. It is our hope that the psychological issues—both theoretical and applied—discussed throughout the book will lead to the enhancement of studying, consulting, and coaching elite athletes.

References

Bloom, B. S. (Ed.). (1985). *Developing talent in young people.* New York: Ballantine Books.

Bompa, T. (1999). *Periodization: The theory and methodology of training* (4th ed.). Champaign, IL: Human Kinetics.

Côté, J., Lidor, R., & Hackfort, D. (in press). To sample or to specialize? —Seven postulates about youth sport activities that lead to continued participation and elite performance. *International Journal of Sport and Exercise Psychology.*

Fisher, R. J., & Borms, J. (1990). *The search for sporting excellence.* Schorndorf: Verlag Karl Hofmann.

Hackfort, D. (2006). A conceptual framework and fundamental issues for investigating the development of peak performance in sports. In D. Hackfort & G. Tenenbaum (Eds.), *Essential processes for attaining peak performance* (pp. 10-25). Oxford: Meyer & Meyer Sport.

Hemery, D. (1986). *Sporting excellence—A study of sport's highest achievers.* Champaign, IL: Human Kinetics.

Howe, M. J. A. (1999). *The psychology of high abilities.* London: Macmillan.

Johnson, M. B., & Tenenbaum, G. (2006). The roles of nature and nurture in expertise in sport. In D. Hackfort & G. Tenenbaum (Eds.), *Essential processes for attaining peak performance* (pp. 26-52). Oxford: Meyer & Meyer Sport.

Kalinowsky, A. G. (1985a). The development of Olympic swimmers. In B. S. Bloom (Ed.), *Developing talent in young people* (pp. 139-192). New York: Ballantine Books.

Kalinowsky, A. G. (1985b). One Olympic swimmer. In B. S. Bloom (Ed.), *Developing talent in young people* (pp. 193-210). New York: Ballantine Books.

Lidor, R., Blumenstein, B., & Tenenbaum, G. (2007). Periodization and planning of psychological preparation in individual and team sports. In B. Blumenstein, R. Lidor, & G. Tenenbaum (Eds.), *Psychology of sport training* (pp. 137-161). London: Meyer & Meyer Sport.

Lidor, R., Côté, J., & Hackfort, D. (in press). To test or not to test?—The use of physical skill tests in talent detection and in early phases of sport development. *International Journal of Sport and Exercise Psychology.*

Monsaas, J. A. (1985). Learning to be a world-class tennis player. In B. S. Bloom (Ed.), *Developing talent in young people* (pp. 211-269). New York: Ballantine Books.

Orlick, T. (2000). *In pursuit of excellence—How to win in sport and life through mental training* (2nd ed.). Champaign, IL: Human Kinetics.

Schilling, G., & Herren, K. (Eds.). (1985). *Excellence and emotional states in sport*. Magglingen: Switzerland.

Singer, R. N., & Janelle, C. M. (1999). Determining sport expertise: From genes to supremes. *International Journal of Sport Psychology, 30,* 117-150.

Vernacchia, R., McGuire, R., & Cook, D. (1992). *Coaching mental excellence: "It does matter whether you win or lose...."* Dubuque, IA: Wm. C. Brown.

CHAPTER 2

The Action Theory-Based Mental Test and Training System (MTTS)

DIETER HACKFORT, CONOR KILGALLEN, AND LIU HAO

The application of sport psychology in elite sports requires (1) the search, identification, and selection of sporting talent; (2) performance enhancement through mental training, mental preparation, and learning strategies; and (3) consultations to ensure the athlete's mental stability in competitive situations and ability to cope with conflicts and crises. These tasks demand a professional, systematic approach based on information derived from diagnostic tools. Modern diagnostic tools utilize computer systems for processing and analyzing data from written assessments, and, more frequently, for providing computerized tests with special features that check performance in various mental processes and domains. Although numerous tests and tools are available, a comprehensive framework is still lacking, and consequently, most of the tests and tools do not have a conceptual-based relation to the appropriate training programs.

The purpose of this chapter is to introduce and report on the development of a Mental Test and Training System (MTTS), which integrates computer-assisted tools with field setups for the testing and training of mental processes and skills deemed important in elite sports. A special emphasis is given to performance-oriented tasks. First, the theoretical background of the MTTS will be outlined.

Theoretical Background of the MTTS

The fundamental idea of the MTTS and the diagnostic and training program is to create a specific action situation—to coordinate the person, the task, and the environment (see Hackfort, 1986) and to modify this constellation for diagnostic or training purposes.

The constellation (see Figure 1) can be altered by referring to the person and modifying, for example, mood states, stress, and cognitive and motivational processes. The state of the person can be modified systematically by influencing existing mental or physical strain or by the announcement (anticipation) of an upcoming stressor. Mental tasks, such as detecting figures or signals, and motor tasks, such as tracking or aiming, can be presented individually or in combination. Reaction

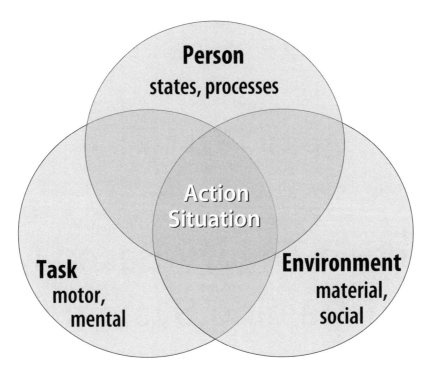

Figure 1. The action situation as the framework for the MTTS.

time measurements are an example of a setup using such combinations. The environment can be modified with respect to, for example, light, noise, temperature, or the presence of (disturbing or facilitating) or absence of (supportive or debilitating) other people. The specific constellation can be used for testing purposes while varying combinations of the above influencing agents can be used for training purposes.

As mental and motor activities are closely interrelated, and the subjective perception and appraisal of the given (objective) circumstances and task at hand are decisive for the organization and regulation (control) of the actions needed to cope with the situation, a multi-method, multi-faceted approach is required for an appropriate strategy to analyze and modify actions. Following this understanding, we use the computer to present tasks, measure performance, and collect and analyze data. We also refer to observations and verbal reports to round off the information for appropriate interpretation of the action processes and results. Both information and the impression of the performance process, as well as the performance outcome, are considered in the test evaluation and the design of training strategies and/or recommendations for practice and competition.

Technical Description of the MTTS

The MTTS is an ongoing developing system that is composed of a mental test system and a mental training system. The main structure of the MTTS is presented in Figure 2.

Both the mental test and the mental training systems consist of a series of computerized/computer-assisted programs as well as field tests and training programs. Features and details of the MTTS will be introduced in the following paragraphs. We will also refer to strategies using a multi-method approach for data collection and for a multi-faceted approach to the interpretation and design of consequences (training, practice).

Computerized Mental Test and Training Systems

Test System

The platform and hardware of the computerized mental test system is based on the Vienna Test System (VTS), which was developed with a focus on clinical and traffic psychology according to the most advanced standards by the Dr. Schuhfried Company located in Vienna,

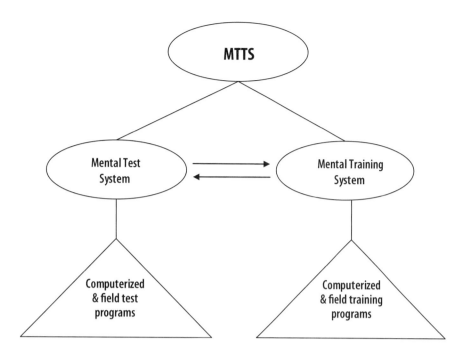

Figure 2. Structure of the MTTS.

Austria. Figure 3 demonstrates the main devices of the system. It is composed of the control unit (for the test administrator) and the action unit (for the client). The control unit is a desktop or laptop computer containing programs of the system, which is manipulated by the test administrator to control the processes of various tests. The action unit includes (1) output devices such as client monitor, peripheral display, flicker and fusion device, and psycho-motor device, by which the instructions and tasks of various tests are presented to the client, and (2) input devices such as client panel, light pen, foot pedals, and so on, by which the client responds to the tasks in various tests.

The system includes various general psycho-motor tests, which are relevant to the performance tests (e.g., reaction time test, two-hand coordination test, peripheral perception test, etc.) and to personality, attitude/interest tests (e.g., Eysenck-Personality-Profiler-V6, Attitude Towards Work, etc.), as well as sport(s)-specific tests that are currently under development by the sport psychology team at ASPIRE Academy for Sports Excellence, Qatar. The Movement Detection Test (BDT) is an example of a sport-specific test aimed at measuring the ability to detect and differentiate movements—an ability that is quite important in a broad variety of sports. The task of the test is to react to the movement of

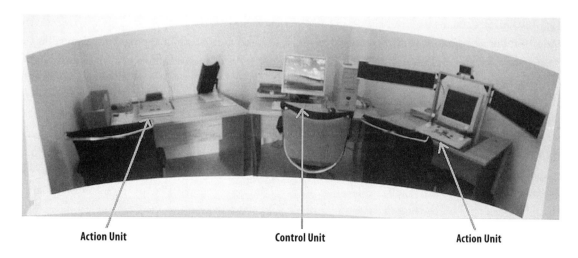

Figure 3. Illustration of the hardware of the mental test system.

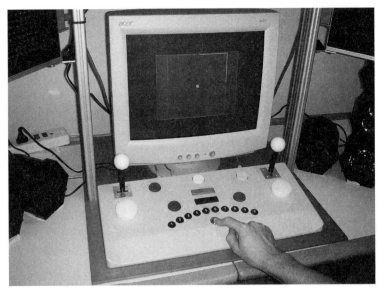

Figure 4. Illustration of the Movement Detection Test (BDT).

a dot in the center of a square on the client monitor. The dot moves randomly from the center to one corner of the square, corresponding to the movement direction. A different button has to be pressed as quickly as possible when the client detects the movements (see Figure 4).

When running the test system, results (various performance indicators/data) can be presented immediately after the test is completed, and can be saved automatically in the database. By using the "find" function, the result of any test conducted on a client can be obtained from the database whenever it is required for individual diagnosis. The system also offers a "data export" function, by which the result of a test conducted on a group of clients can be converted into a SPSS file for research.

Training System

The organization of mental training, which includes developing training situations, is one of the two broad domains of mental training (Hackfort, 2001). The development of the mental training system in the frame of the MTTS is based on this understanding of and approach to mental training, and the fundamental idea of the system is to create various action situations for training purposes. The computerized mental training system is a combination of mental test system tasks and a specific setup to cope with the tasks, that is, the creation of special training situations. According to the action theory-based approach on mental training (e.g., Hackfort, 1986; Hackfort & Munzert, 2005; Nitsch & Hackfort, 1981), a training situation is a special action situation re-

garded as a person-environment-task constellation (see Figure 5). The person is related to the physical and/or mental state of the client during the training, the task is related to the format and/or complexity of task in the training, and the environment refers to training environment, which includes both material and social environments. Various training situations can be created by modifying this constellation.

Figure 6 is an illustration of two training situations created in the computerized mental training system. In Figure 6a, a bicycle is used to create a motion situation, which is integrated with a Peripheral Perception Test (PPT) for training purposes. In the training process, the client has to synchronously respond to the PPT and ride the bicycle under varying levels of physical load. Riding the bicycle creates a new training situation in which the client's physical state is changed and the complexity of the task is increased. Training in such situations is designed to effectively improve the client's peripheral perception. In Figure 6b, disturbing lights are used to modify the training environment, and these can be integrated with all the performance tests for training purposes. In addition to the cycle and the disturbing lights, CDs with various noises (e.g., white noise, noise of spectators in a sports competition) can also be used to create different training situations. These three training situations can be used separately, or the elements can be combined in different ways to create further training situations.

Another important element of the computerized mental training system is a wireless biofeedback system.

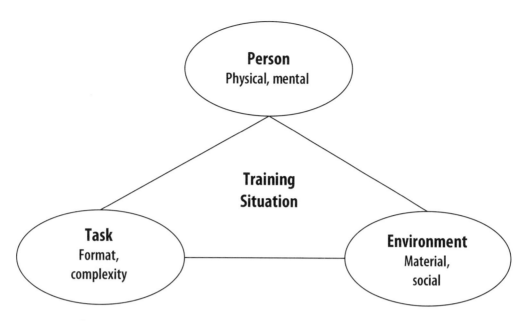

Figure 5. Training situation as a special person-environment-task constellation.

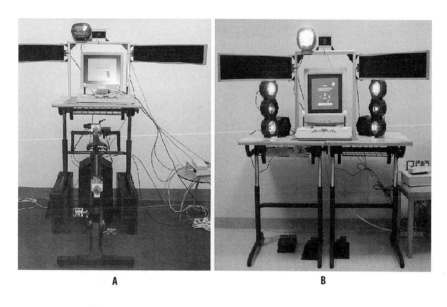

A   B

Figure 6. Two setups in the computerized training system.

The hardware of the biofeedback system from the Dr. Schuhfried Company includes: (1) a desktop or laptop with biofeedback programs, (2) one client monitor connected to the desktop or laptop, and (3) three radio modules. The first module has three different sensors that record temperature feedback (TEMP), pulse amplitude and frequency feedback (PULS), and skin conductance (EDA) separately. The second module can be used to analyze the client's breathing pattern and to compare abdominal and thoracic breathing, if it is connected with an add-on module for these purposes. The third module can be connected to two 2-pole and one 1-pole electrode cables in order to measure muscle tension. With wireless design, the long cables leading to a central unit for signal transmission are replaced by radio modules. Only very short sensor cables are needed to pass the signal from the sensors to the radio modules, which prevent the feeling of being wired. During the training session the client receives visual and acoustic feedback on his or her physiological reactions. Various feedback options are available in the system.

Biofeedback training in combination with cognitive strategies can be used to create a new training situation in order to learn how to monitor the psycho-physiological

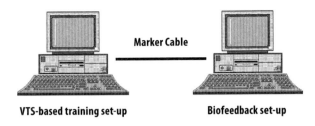

Marker Cable

VTS-based training set-up   Biofeedback set-up

Figure 7. Linking of systems.

state. The development of cognitive strategies for respiration control with the assistance of the biofeedback equipment is a good application of biofeedback tools in the computerized mental training system. The whole training program consists of three steps:

(1) Introduction of the basic concept of deep abdominal breathing for relaxation purposes, as well as the basic method of deep abdominal breathing;

(2) Elaboration on strategies and training of deep abdominal breathing with the biofeedback system. The respiration training program in the biofeedback system can be used specifically for abdominal breathing training. At the beginning of the training session, the client is asked to breathe deeply several times using the abdominal style. The computer then analyzes the client's breathing pattern and immediately calculates an ideal respiration curve and displays the curve on the screen. After that, the client is asked to start his or her breathing training and to determine an appropriate strategy resulting in a fit with the ideal respiration curve;

(3) Mental training in the computerized system. The client is asked to start a training session assisted by the system, following the abdominal breathing training. It is assumed that the relaxed state after the breathing training will improve the subsequent training effectiveness.

In addition, the biofeedback can be linked to VTS-based training by a marker cable (see Figure 7). This connection makes it possible to record physiological data during the training period, and to determine the optimal physiological state corresponding to a peak performance.

For example, the EMG value of the client's arm can be recorded during several training sessions and then analyzed to determine the optimal value for peak performance. This value can then be used as a threshold in future training sessions.

Field Test and Training System

As with the computerized mental test and training systems, a field test and training system is also under ongoing development. At ASPIRE, the applied sport psychology staff strives to build on participants' learning from the computerized testing and training by challenging participants in other areas. A setup and sequence of computerized MTTS → practical/virtual laboratory → field training has been established. Testing and training on the computerized MTTS and in the practical/virtual labs has proved to be a very enjoyable, efficient, and safe way of learning mental skills and strategies before attempting them in real sport. Virtual sports games and practical lab games such as motor slot racing are examples of fun yet challenging ways of transferring learning from the computerized MTTS, and can even lead to the development of additional mental strategies.

In addition to furthering mental training in a different environment, practical lab tests are ideal ways of validating tests done on the computerized MTTS. A good example of this is a lab tool (game), named Action-Check, created and designed by ASPIRE's sport psychology team. The "game" is essentially a cross between several ball sports (e.g., football, bowling, basketball, golf-putting), and its purpose is to assess a combination of achievement motivation and risk-taking behavior. The link between achievement motivation and risk-taking (both of which can be assessed on the computerized MTTS and by the Action-Check) is significant. Reference will be given to the theories behind the tests and the subsequent development of the lab game.

Risk Choice, also known by the test label RISIKO, is a test on the computerized MTTS for assessment of general readiness to take risks. Readiness to take risks describes a global style of behavior in respect to which differences between individuals can be identified (Andresen, 1995; Schwenkmezger, 1988). Based on the Risk Choice Model (Atkinson, 1957), one's overall readiness for risk-taking is assessed in RISIKO by examining achievement motivation, as exposure to real risk for experimental purposes cannot be ethically justified. Achievement motivation in general is the need that drives an individual to improve, succeed, or excel. The test itself consists of a moving ball on the screen, which undergoes unpredictable changes in direction. The participant's task is to use a control lever to create a circle that encloses the ball and to keep the ball within the circle. Points are scored for keeping the ball within the circle. The aim is to score as many points as possible. The participant chooses the radius size before each run. A smaller radius can potentially lead to more points being scored but the risk is higher as the task becomes harder with a decrease in radius size. The test is made up of four phases, with different conditions in each phase: (a) ball moves slowly, (b) ball moves fast, (c) control of circle is rotated counter-clockwise by 90 degrees, and (d) conditions of the first three phases occur apparently at random.

The Risk Choice Model examines factors that influence the selection of the level of a challenge. Atkinson (1957) assumes that one acts in accordance with the probability of being able to cope with the selected level of difficulty. The easier the task, the greater is the probability of success. However, people also strive for challenges. The level of challenge describes what an individual intends to do (Rheinberg, 1997). Furthermore, difficulty of a task is always subjective (Rheinberg). An extremely difficult task has a very high incentive for success; however, realistically, achievement motivation is very low, as the probability of success is close to zero. Likewise, achievement motivation is equally low in the case of simplified tasks, where there is a 100 % certainty of accomplishment.

In addition to having an intensity aspect, the Risk Choice Model also assumes that achievement motivation has a direction component; that is, whether a person anticipates and organizes his or her actions for probable success or to prevent failure when facing a task. Thus, individuals can be described as either "success-approaching oriented" or "failure-avoidance oriented." In brief, success-approaching oriented individuals prefer moderately high goals. Therefore, they choose an open and undetermined outcome of which they have a high probability of being able to influence through the exercise of their skill (Otti, 1993). Their approach to goal setting is flexible and takes into account current performance and the associated prospects of success. In contrast, failure-avoidance oriented individuals set goals that are either so low that they are almost certain to be achieved, or so

high that they would be unattainable for most people. Following failure, such people stick to pre-determined goals and do not take the current performance level and associated prospects of success into account. Their approach to goal setting, therefore, is rigid.

While achievement motivation is examined in RISIKO for the purpose of assessing readiness to take risks, another computerized MTTS test, the Objective Achievement Motivation Test (OLMT), examines achievement motivation in a different way. The OLMT provides information on the effort put into working the test under various significant motivating conditions. It consists of three subtests, each of which is built around a particular incentive or stimulus that is relevant to motivating respondents' performance: incentives arising from the task itself, from setting one's own goals, and from competition. The task in each subtest is simply to cover as much ground in a "route" as possible in ten seconds, by pressing appropriate buttons for moving left or right.

In both OLMT and RISIKO, there is an opportunity for the test administrator to observe the participant's intentional organized behavior. Useful information can be gathered on the approaches to goal setting (see, e.g., Weinberg & Butt, 2005). It is also useful to observe tactical, physical, and mental strategies employed by participants for improving or for striving to reach a target. This information can later be used in making participants aware of their behavior, and when necessary, it can form the basis of advice recommending more efficient strategies. Moreover, the use of a DVD camcorder for immediate visual feedback has proven to be popular and informative among test participants for increasing their awareness of existing behavior and for the explanation of action organization, action control, and recommendations for modifications by the psychologist.

While RISIKO and OLMT provide valuable information on readiness to take risks and achievement motivation, respectively, Action-Check was specially developed for combining the best elements of both tests and to serve as a means of validating the results. As already mentioned, this lab task is designed to mimic several ball sports. The task is to kick (or throw, or roll) a ball into a hole. As illustrated in Figure 8, the hole is situated on a raised platform. The goal of successfully kicking the ball into the hole is attainable but challenging. The greater the distance is between ball and hole, the more difficult the task.

Action-Check is a tool under ongoing development,

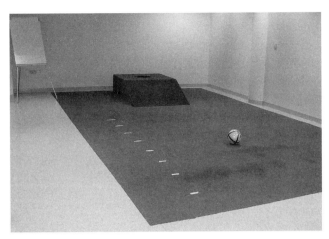

Figure 8. Action-Check.

with continual improvements being sought in regard to rules and interpretations of the concept of action (intentional organized behavior). At the time of writing this chapter, special rules are in place for assessing readiness to take risks and also for assessing the intensity and direction of achievement motivation. A set of rules for the "game" were agreed upon based on the Risk Choice Model (Atkinson, 1957). The objective of the task, as far as the participants are concerned, is to score as many points as possible. The participant has a choice of where to shoot from. As seen in Figure 8, there are eight white strips on the left side of the green carpet, each 45 centimeters apart. Shots must be taken from a point level with one of these strips. The strip closest to the hole provides a score of +1 for a successful shot or -1 for a miss. For each strip one moves away from the hole, one can score an extra point, but also potentially lose an extra point for a miss. Therefore, the strip farthest from the hole, which represents the greatest challenge or risk, provides scores of +8 or -8, depending on the success of the shot. To make the game more strategic and risk-laden, participants start with a 20-point credit. If they reach zero at any point, they are disqualified. So, for example, three consecutive misses from the start at the 7-point strip will cause disqualification. Therefore, the risk of going for higher points is tactically, as well as practically, greater.

In practice, Action-Check provides an excellent opportunity for observing intentional organized behavior (actions). Firstly, one can observe any changes in behavior, from a pre-task familiarization exercise to the exercise itself. Secondly, one can observe from the sequence in the strategy of selecting starting positions, along with the success of the shots (i.e., flexibility of goal-setting), whether their achievement motivation is high or low,

whether they are success-approaching or failure-avoidance oriented, and whether their readiness to take risks is high or low. Furthermore, variety can be introduced into this lab game. For example, as with the OLMT, one can observe how participants intentionally behave under different motivating conditions. That is, one can compare or contrast the behavior of an individual when in a competitive situation with other participants when he or she is doing the task alone, and when setting his or her own goals. Additionally, if monitoring competitive behavior, it is worth asking participants in which order they would like to compete (e.g., first, second, last). Information gleaned from this may provide further indications about participants' achievement motivation. For example, one could argue that by choosing to go first, the participant is not easily influenced by competitors' actions. Instead, the participant chooses to focus on his or her own performance, a possible indicator of a success-approaching orientation. If, for example, a participant immediately chooses to go last, it might indicate the existence of strategic intentions that will focus specifically on observations of the competitors' actions. Depending on the flexibility of goals in this scenario, one could make a case that the participant is either success-approaching- or failure-avoidance-oriented.

The link between the aforementioned computerized MTTS tests (RISIKO and OLMT) and the specially-built Action-Check is one example of the ASPIRE sport psychology team's approach to transferring learning and training from one setting to another. The lab task also serves to validate the MTTS tests. Meanwhile, another example of a popular practical lab tool used for mental training purposes is an advanced motor slot racing game (see Figure 9). This will now be discussed briefly.

The motor slot racing game has proved to be an exciting addition to the ASPIRE sport psychology unit's practical lab. The task of completing a lap on the race track in good time requires acute reaction times, concentration, and emotional control. Again, this tool fits in nicely in the environmental sequence: computerized MTTS → practical/virtual lab → field. In the first stage of this sequence, as mentioned previously, mental strategies are taught and trained depending on the situation. For example, participants may benefit from advice on mental and physical pre-task preparation, or perhaps from cognitive strategies for improving concentration and overcoming mistakes. It is strongly encouraged that lessons learned during the computer-assisted element of training be used in training on the motor slot racing (practical lab task).

The motor slot racing tool is also an excellent way of introducing imagery in a practical way (Hackfort & Munzert, 2005; Schack, 2004; Schack & Hackfort, 2007). In a training scenario, participants are required to build up a mental representation of the track and focus on the rhythm with the intention of being able to complete laps afterwards with their vision occluded. An example of a task on the slot racing track with vision occluded is ten timed trials to complete ten laps without crashing or stopping. When the visual sense is absent, the participant has to compensate by heightening other senses (e.g., hearing the car, touching the control) and blending this information with a sense of lap timing to create a perfect rhythm. Evidence from trials to date with this training approach suggests that such an internal-focused and process-oriented approach to training can produce sharpened performance outcomes when final testing (the same design as training) is done with the eyes open. While improved performance on a slot racing game is not the most important objective of mental training, the raw time figures from the lap counter serve to "convince" the participant of the success of their chosen mental strategies. The message from this lab training is then to take and apply this new learning in real-life sport (the final step in the sequence: computerized MTTS → practical/virtual lab → field).

Summary

At present, computer and other relevant technologies are playing an increasing role in sport diagnosis and training. The MTTS, based on an action-theory concept, includes a computerized mental test system and a computerized mental training system. The fundamental idea is to create specific person-task-environment constellations as action situations for testing and training purposes. In the computerized mental test system, the performance-oriented tests, which require the client to respond to various special tasks by pressing button(s) and/or foot pedal(s), can provide more accurate performance-relevant information than traditional paper-and-pencil inventories, and the utility of mental strategies (e.g., imagery, deep breathing, and muscle relaxation) can be observed directly during the test. The computerized mental training system, conceptually, is a combination of tasks of the mental test system and the creation

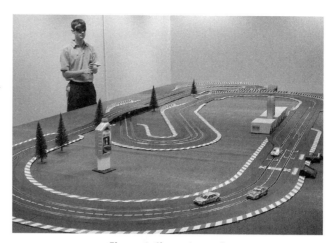

Figure 9. Slot racing task.

of special training situations. By modifying the person-task-environment constellation, a series of highly individualized and sport(s)-specific training programs can be tailored. In the process of training, various mental skills such as imagery, relaxation, and self-talk, as well as mental preparation, are learned. This new learning is further tried and developed in the practical/virtual lab (e.g., slot racing), and then, ultimately, the field (i.e., real-life sport). This sequence of mental training is currently being used by the authors with student-athletes at the ASPIRE Academy for Sports Excellence in Doha, Qatar. Specially-tailored training programs in the framework of this approach have already been developed for some elite sports (e.g., Formula One racing and squash). Subjective feedback from participants on such programs reveals a feeling of a decrease in effort/energy for the same or improved performance. Objective test results from post-training testing support this positive feedback with evidence of improved performances on specific tests. Likewise, observation during final testing can confirm whether or not newly-learned mental strategies are employed.

MTTS is an ongoing developing system. At present, work on further tools for testing and training purposes is in progress.

References

Andresen, B. (1995). Risikobereitschaft (R)—der sechste Basisfaktor der Personlichkeit: Konvergenz multivariater Studien und Konstruktexplikation [Risk taking (R)—the sixth basis factor of personality: Convergence of multivariate studies and construct explication.]. *Zeitschrift fur Differentielle und Diagnostiche Psychologie, 16*, 210-236.

Atkinson, J. W. (1957). Motivational determinants of risk-taking behavior. *Psychological Review, 64*, 359-372.

Hackfort, D. (1986). *Theorie und Analyse sportbezogener Ängstlichkeit* [Theory and analysis of sport-related trait anxiety]. Schorndorf, Germany: Hofmann.

Hackfort, D. (2001). Experiences with application of Action-Theory-Based Approach in working with elite athletes. In G. Tenenbaum (Ed.), *The practice of sport psychology* (pp. 89-100). Morgantown, WV: Fitness Information Technology.

Hackfort, D., & Munzert, J. (2005). Mental simulation. In D. Hackfort, J. Duda, & R. Lidor (Eds.), *Handbook of research in applied sport and exercise psychology—International perspectives* (pp. 3-16). Morgantown, WV: Fitness Information Technology.

Nitsch, J. R., & Hackfort, D. (1981). *Streß in Schule und Hochschule—eine handlungspsychologische Funktionsanalyse* [Stress at school and university: A functional analysis based on action theory]. In J. R. Nitsch (Ed.), *Stress. Theorien, Untersuchungen, Maßnahmen* (pp. 263-311). Bern, Switzerland: Huber.

Otti, A. (1993). *Ergopsychometrie. Leistungsmotivation und Handgeschicklichkeit als Moderatorvariablen der Risikobereitschaft [Ergopsychometry. Achievement motivation and manual skill as a moderator variable of risk taking.)*. Unveroffentliche Diplomarbeit (Unpublished diploma thesis), Universitaet Wien.

Rheinberg, F. (1997). *Motivation (2. und uberarbeitete Auflage)* [Motivation, 2nd ed.]. Stuttgart, Berlin, Koeln: Kohlhammer.

Schack, T. (2004). Relation of knowledge and performance in motor action. *Journal of Knowledge Management, 4,* 38-53.

Schack, T., & Hackfort, D. (2007). Action-theory approach to applied sport psychology. In G. Tenenbaum & R. C. Eklund (Eds.), *Handbook of sport psychology* (3rd ed., pp. 332-351). Hoboken, NJ: Wiley.

Schwenkmezger, P. (1988). Der Risikobegriff der Psychologie: Definitionen, Theorien, Erfassungsmethoden [The concept of risk in psychology: Definitions, theories, measurements]. In P. Compes (Hrsg.), *Risiko—subjektiv und objektiv.* IX Internationales Sommer-Symposium: Mainz.

Weinberg, R., & Butt, J. (2005). Goal setting in sport and exercise domains: The theory and practice of effective goal setting. In D. Hackfort, J. L. Duda, & R. Lidor (Eds.), *Handbook of research in applied sport and exercise psychology—International perspectives* (pp. 129-144). Morgantown, WV: Fitness Information Technology.

CHAPTER 3

A Sport Psychology Service Delivery Model for Developing and Current Track and Field Athletes and Coaches

TRACI STATLER AND KEITH HENSCHEN

This chapter, divided into two distinct parts, will introduce and describe a model of sport psychology service delivery available to track and field athletes in the United States. The first part of this chapter will introduce sport psychology practitioners, coaches, and athletes to the short-term, intensive education program presented each summer to some of America's best developing youth track and field athletes. The goal of this chapter is to share a popular and effective sport psychology consulting model with those seeking an understanding of how to initiate and integrate a sport psychology program with potential Olympians. The second portion of the chapter will then describe how this developmental foundation is fostered as the athlete continues to progress, eventually emerging at the elite rank of "Olympian" or "World Champion."

The authors will explain the guiding purpose and general educational mission of the USA Track & Field (USATF) sport psychology program, which has been an integral part of the development of American track

and field athletes since the program's inception in 1982. Conducted by highly experienced practitioners in the field of sport psychology, it has served to "promote and deliver sport psychology services through coaching education programs, camps, clinics, workshops, team travel, and educational writings" (Vernacchia & Statler, 2005, p. 5).

Sport Psychology for the Developing Track and Field Athlete

Developing American track and field athletes often learn about the benefits of sport psychology when they are invited to attend a USATF-sponsored Junior Elite Camp. These camps, held at U.S. Olympic Training Centers, aim to inspire and aid in the development of elite high school athletes and their coaches toward international, and eventually, Olympic-level participation. Close to 5,000 athletes and coaches have progressed though these intensive camps, and many current Olympians and World Champions count themselves as alumni of this program.

The dynamics and organization of the USATF Junior Elite Camps are carefully defined in an effort to produce the greatest overall improvements in existing performance in the shortest amount of time. These programs, running a mere one week in duration, are incredibly intensive and address all elements of competition from technique and physical conditioning to nutritional needs and sport psychology. Several camps are scheduled each summer, each focusing on a specific event group in track and field, so as to specifically target the training methods best suited to each athlete's required skill set. For athletes and coaches, this intensive mini-camp is often the first experience with applying sport psychology skills to their performance.

A typical day's schedule at one of these camps includes a combination of classroom-setting workshops and on-track, hands-on experiential sessions. The workshops cover such topics as "Nutrition for Elite Sprinters," "The Importance and Physiology of Speed, Quickness, Strength, Power, and Dynamic Flexibility Development of Throwers," and "Sport Psychology Skills and Interventions for Relay Athletes and Their Coaches." The track-based sessions include elements such as "Speed and Quickness Training Activities" for each specific event group, and field testing and skill evaluation sessions. The typical day's activities begin by 7:00 am, continuing throughout the day and ending at 10:00 pm, when the athletes return to their dorm rooms to rest and prepare for the next day's activities.

Introduction to Sport Psychology

During the first full day of these camps, the athletes and their coaches are introduced to a sport psychology specialist assigned to their event camp. During that first introductory session, the athletes are given a brief overview followed by a series of psychometric inventories that serve as a starting point for personalized, one-on-one discussions to follow later. These inventories include the State-Trait Anxiety Inventory (STAI) (Spielberger, Gorsuch, & Lushene, 1970); a modified and shortened version of the Test of Attentional and Interpersonal Style (TAIS) (Nideffer, 1989); and the Achievement Motivation Scale for Supporting Environments (AMSSE) (Rushall & Fox, 1980). The athletes complete these inventories on the first night and submit them back to the

sport psychology consultant to be scored and evaluated prior to the next day's session. We have found that using this method on the first night allows the consultant to develop an initial understanding of each individual athlete, which can then be used to inform and direct more personalized discussions. Furthermore, this creates an opportunity to foster a beginning level of trust between the athlete and the sport psychology consultant, which in many cases continues to develop throughout the course of the athlete's career.

Sport Psychology Educational Modules
As mentioned earlier, participants in these Junior Camps will have a variety of classroom sessions with various experts on different elements of sport science. For the sessions on sport psychology and performance enhancement, four specific training modules are presented. These modules are designed to interactively educate less-experienced participants on a personal performance level in the areas of motivation, arousal and anxiety management, concentration skills, and imagery for enhanced performance. The idea behind educating participants in these specific areas is that the mental skill set required to achieve elite performance clearly includes these elements. Furthermore, as will be explained in the second part of this chapter, these skills serve as foundational components of additional education and frequently come up in performance consultations later in the athletes' elite development. Though these sessions are presented in an educational, classroom-type setting, the actual interaction allows the athletes, as well as their parents and coaches, to personalize the content and tailor it to their own individual performance.

The content of these modules is very similar to an introductory sport psychology class, though with more of a primary emphasis on personal application and less on theoretical foundations underlying the skill's effectiveness. In the module on motivation, the discussion centers on the inherent benefits and drawbacks of intrinsic and extrinsic motivators, and the difference between the motive to succeed versus the motive to avoid failure. Again, the discussion is tailored to personal application, so elucidating how these factors manifest themselves in practice and performance settings is critical. In the module on anxiety and arousal regulation, the discussion centers on the differences between state and trait anxiety, and on techniques for improved management of performance anxiety. The concentration module centers on developing an understanding of the typical distractors these athletes face, as well as providing tools for limiting personal distractions and for building training-appropriate focus. Lastly, the module on the use of imagery for performance improvement typically generates a discussion of the uses and benefits of effective imagery and gives guidelines for incorporating it into practice and performance settings.

By the conclusion of these training camps, these developing athletes and their coaches and parents will have spent several days interacting with the sport psychologist, and most leave the experience with a greater understanding of how sport psychology can be used to improve performance, both on and off the track. It is common for an athlete we have met with at one of these developmental camps to re-emerge as a member of a U.S. traveling team (i.e., Junior or Senior Pan American Games, World Championships, international dual meets, Olympics, etc.) sometime later in their career. As they confront the demands of elite-level national or international competition, these athletes are better equipped to receive psychological services due to the foundational and educational introduction at the training camps. The athletes are familiar with the services we as sport psychology consultants can provide, they generally feel more comfortable approaching the sport psychologist for assistance, and they have already had some experience with practicing the mental skills necessary for enhancing performance.

Service Delivery for the Elite and Olympic Athlete

The first portion of this chapter outlined what is offered to the developing track and field athlete, and now the second portion will articulate the programs that are available to the Olympic/elite athletes.

The national organizing committee for track and field in the United States currently has 18 applied sport psychology consultants who service the sport of track and field in all programs overseen by this organization. These 18 professionals were carefully evaluated prior to their inclusion in this Track and Field Sport Psychology Group. Only certain types of applied sport psychology consultants have the complementary service-delivery philosophy, past experiences, and the demonstrated personality characteristics to be included in this group. This group of consultants is very diverse, in order to

meet all the different functions it is asked to facilitate for the USATF organization. We consider gender, ethnic background, athletic experience, educational background—clinical or applied, and previous demonstrated competencies. Each person who is invited to join the group undergoes a mentoring process. He or she will be invited (usually two per year) to the National Championships for 3-4 days of mentoring from the Executive Committee. This mentoring consists of discussions about the group's philosophy, do's and don'ts concerning working with elite athletes, and the general responsibilities of members of the group. Many sport psychologists have asked to join this group, but only a few are eventually included. Fitting into the sport psychology group is imperative because its members are very closeknit. Again, these sport psychologists are very accomplished in their own right, but they must be willing and able to abide by the group's philosophy and procedures to maintain its integrity in track and field.

The individual sport psychologists working in this group are located in cities and towns across the United States, so that no matter where the athletes reside, they will have sport psychology services readily available any time during the year. Also, any time a track and field team (junior or senior) travels or competes internationally representing the United States, two members of the sport psychology group are assigned to accompany the team as part of the staff. Normally, one of these two professionals is credentialed as a clinical sport psychologist and the other is an experienced applied sport psychology consultant. Because the track teams representing the United States are composed of both male and female athletes, we also attempt to send both a male and a female sport psychology consultant as part of the traveling staff.

In addition to traveling, the sport psychology consultants are also intricately involved in elite-level coaching clinics and high-performance athlete clinics throughout the year. These types of involvement are presented for the sole purpose of illustrating that sport psychology services are continual, extensive, and viewed as an important part of the sports medicine services provided for our promising and elite athletes. This chapter provides both an overview and the practical applications of various aspects of the service delivery framework that is utilized during the Olympics and throughout the quadrennium that precedes the games.

Service Delivery Philosophy

No matter which members of the sports psychology group are eventually assigned to work with the Olympic team, we have all adopted a similar philosophy, which is an educational approach to performance enhancement in international settings. While group interventative approaches are used at times (infrequently), the vast majority of the interventions with coaches and athletes, before and during the Olympic Games, falls into the category of "conversational" sport psychology. In other words, services are delivered at one-on-one consulting sessions and in predominately informal circumstances. This "spur of the moment" delivery of services is effective because the athlete needs something that will immediately work. If the consultant can provide little techniques that are useful, then an opportunity is opened for more detailed work in the future. It is rather unusual to have the time (at the Games) to teach lasting skill development, but credibility will be enhanced if the consultant can provide innovative methods in the short run that overcome problems. The times to do this are on the practice fields, at meal time, and even during transportation to and from practices or competitions. These are the kind of interactions that build rapport and/or break down inhibitions.

Mental Skills Training

By the time an athlete reaches a high level of physical skill, the natural assumption is that he or she has also mastered a set of accompanying psychological skills. This is a false assumption—at least in the United States. The reality is that many experienced athletes have become reliant on sheer physical prowess. Frequently, the mental skills are either lacking or in their infancy. The mental skills training performed with Olympic athletes is then based upon individual needs, and seems to occur primarily in three areas: (1) Composure, (2) Attention control, and (3) Confidence (Vernacchia & Statler, 2005).

Composure Training

As the Olympic Games approach, emotional pressure, both real and perceived, intensifies for the athletes and coaches. It should be the sport psychology consultants' objective to help the athletes and coaches feel comfortable in normally uncomfortable situations by teaching them how to respond effectively to the stresses and pressures they are about to experience. Emotional compo-

sure is essential to delivering—on demand—world-class track and field performances at World Championships and Olympic Games, and this composure should not be dissipated by doubt, fear, or anxiety.

The emotional distractions and challenges the athletes face prior to, during, and even after the Olympic Games are enormous, and a great deal of personal control is required to cope with these issues in a healthy and productive manner. During world-class competitions, the performance environment is changing constantly, and athletes must demonstrate passive willpower (patience) in order to keep focused and on target, and more effective. This is a difficult skill for an elite athlete who has become one of the best in the world through physical prowess and hard work. Therefore, it is critical that they learn to allow their performances to "flow," rather than trying to "force" them. In essence, the elite performer must "try less" on one of the most important days of his or her career.

The real key to effective performances at high-level competitions is the ability to control excitement or arousal levels. Although elite athletes may experience nervousness or apprehension as their events approach, it is also typical for these highly successful athletes to be excited and ready to showcase their talents to the world. Frequently, at this time, they become impatient, and once again, composure and emotional control are mandatory.

In order to help elite athletes learn how to master the skill of composure, the sport psychology consultants teach these skills (hands on) at the high-performance clinics that were previously mentioned. The skills taught include relaxation, arousal regulation, pressure management, and pre-competition mental routines.

Relaxation and Arousal Regulation. These two concepts appear to exist on opposite ends of a continuum; however, where the one ends and the other begins is very subtle, and individual athletes have unique levels at which they perform optimally. One must be cognizant of the feelings of both of these physiological states to be able to control them. This involves preparation of the mind and the body by establishing the ideal activation level. To accomplish this feat, relaxation training is normally taught initially to reduce excessive levels of anxiety and stress, and then to train the mind to communicate effectively with the feelings of the body. The mind and body listen to each other's signals (Henschen & Straub, 1995). Physical relaxation is based on the principle that arousal and relaxation are opposites and cannot occur simultaneously in the body. As the athlete learns from the skill of relaxation, it becomes possible to monitor desirable levels of arousal (tension) of the body. This entails becoming aware of how activation and/or relaxation feel on many different levels. Eventually, the performer will learn to create the level of relaxation or arousal in order to perform optimally in any situation and at various levels of pressure. Relaxation techniques frequently taught include breathing awareness (Jiang, 1992), progressive relaxation (Jacobsen, 1930), and autogenic training (Krenz, 1983).

Pressure. This phenomenon is a cognitive state that our minds create. Every athlete feels it, but few handle it effectively. There are three ways that athletes can respond to this perceived pressure: (1) by dividing their attention and thus being distracted, (2) by over-analyzing and thus thinking too much, or (3) by viewing the situation as a challenge instead of a threat. Of course, the first two ways impede performance, while the third enhances the ability to perform. Learning to perceive pressure as a challenge is accomplished by mastering the skills of composure, concentration, and confidence. The skill of composure is developed by establishing a pre-competition mental routine; this will be discussed in the confidence section because it overlaps both areas.

Attention Control Training

Sport psychology consultants view concentration as the ability to maintain a clear and present focus. Many of our Olympic athletes have a need for focusing and refocusing strategies because they have difficulty coping with distractions that seem to accompany high-level competitions (e.g., World Championships and Olympic Games). All athletes recognize very quickly that, without appropriate concentration, their performances become inconsistent, erratic, and error prone. Whatever this phenomenon entails, it is obvious that great athletes have it and the less proficient need it. Concentration training should emphasize all of the attentional styles so that they occur automatically as the circumstances demand. The following are attentional styles that all performers should master:

Narrow Internal – A narrow focus on an internal feeling or object.

Broad Internal – Directing attention internally in order to analyze, think about, and deal with a large amount of information.

Narrow External – A narrow focus on an external object or task.

Broad External – Being aware of everything going on around you.

Shifting – The ability to move from one type of attentional style to another very quickly. (Nideffer, 1989)

The skills of concentration are probably the most crucial to actual performance of all performance psychological skills. Athletes are helped to acquire concentration through three techniques: (1) exercises designed to develop each of the attentional styles, (2) attuning, and (3) pre-competitive mental routines. The exercises are presented in Appendix A. Attuning is simply making sure the athletes feel familiar with their surroundings as quickly as possible—becoming attuned to important factors such as the living arrangements, other competitors, actual protocols and time sequences of the competition, the practice and competitive venues, the drug testing facilities, seating arrangements, and location of the staff and coaches during competitions. Many "walk throughs" are conducted so that each athlete can become familiar and somewhat comfortable in all the situations to which he or she could be exposed. The pre-competition mental routine will be discussed in the next section.

Confidence Training

Most athletes have their confidence shaken at various times surrounding the Olympic Games. Actually, this is quite natural because confidence is a state, not a trait. Not only is confidence a state, but it is also extremely fragile in most elite performers. Confidence can be enhanced by mastering a number of psychological skills, such as the previous ones mentioned (e.g., relaxation, concentration) but also some others: imagery, appropriate self-talk, and pre-competition mental routines.

Imagery. Imagery offers a number of possibilities because it allows a focus on important visual cues and physical skills as they unfold in the moment; it functions "like a language for action" (Heil, 1995, p. 183). Often imagery is used synonymously with visualization, but this is incorrect; visualization is only one form of imagery. Most high-level athletes are kinesthetic imagers (feelers), although they still use some visual imagery as well. Imagery is a skill we teach athletes because it enhances performance and contributes to confidence if used properly.

Self-Talk. All of us talk to ourselves. We actually talk to ourselves in our heads using emotional tones as well as words. The tone of this dialogue can affect our behaviors, our emotions, and consequently our physical states. Negative self-talk leads to frustration, anger, anxiety, and depression. Positive self-talk is uplifting and a confidence builder. Self-talk is not an easy thing to change. Again, we have exercises (see Appendix B) that help teach athletes to manage their self-talk in a positive direction in order to help maximize their performance. How we think and talk to ourselves in our minds dictates the direction our body will follow.

Pre-Competition Performance Routines. After learning the psychological skills of relaxation, concentration, imagery, and self-talk, the athlete should be able to use them in a number of ways—for example, in a pre-competition performance routine. Such a routine will enhance the probability of a good and consistent physical performance. A pre-competition mental routine is unique to each individual and should be practiced frequently in order to perfect it and build confidence in it. It should be short (1-2 minutes), use a number of the mental skills already learned, and place the mind in a state where it is ready to allow the body to perform. In other words, this mental routine should allow an athlete to trust his or her training.

In this chapter we attempted to explain how the sport psychology group for the USATF works with the coaches and athletes in this sport. We have programs of sport psychology for developing athletes as well as for those at the elite level. The mental skills training provided by the sport psychology professionals is aimed at helping to prepare the athlete for many of the challenges that he or she will face in training and competition.

References

Heil, J. (1995). Imagery. In K. P. Henschen & W. F. Straub (Eds.), *Sport psychology: An analysis of athlete behavior* (pp. 183-191). Longmeadow, MA: Monument.

Henschen, K. P., & Straub, W. F. (1995). *Sport psychology: An analysis of athlete behavior* (3rd ed.). Longmeadow, MA: Monument.

Jacobsen, E. (1930). *Progressive relaxation.* Chicago: University of Chicago Press.

Jiang, Z. (1992). *The effects of Qi Gong training on postworkout anxiety, mood state, and heart rate recovery of high school swimmers.* Unpublished Doctoral Disseration, University of Utah.

Krenz, E. W. (1983). *Modified autogenic training.* Salt Lake City, UT: L.L.P. Associates.

Nideffer, R. M. (1989). *Attention control training for sport.* San Diego, CA: Educational and Industrial Testing Service.

Reardon. J. P. (1995). Handling the self talk of athletes. In K. P. Henschen & W. F. Straub (Eds.), *Sport psychology: An analysis of athlete behavior* (3rd ed., pp. 203-211). Longmeadow, MA: Monument.

Rushall, B. S., & Fox, R. G. (1980). An approach-avoidance motivation scale for sporting environments. *Canadian Journal of Applied Sport Sciences, 5,* 39-43.

Spielberger, C. D., Gorsuch, R. L., & Lushene, R. E. (1970). *Manual for the State-Trait Anxiety Inventory.* Palo Alto, CA: Consulting Psychologists Press.

Vernacchia, R. A., & Statler, T. A. (2005). *The psychology of high performance track and field.* Mountain View, CA: Track and Field News.

Appendix A

1. **Listening to outside sounds (broad external)**
   Lie down with your eyes closed and just concentrate on the sounds that are occurring around you (3 minutes).

2. **Monitoring the sounds of your body (broad external)**
   Lie on your back with eyes closed and fingers in your ears. Then focus on all the sounds of your body—growling of stomach, breathing, and heartbeat (2 minutes).

3. **Flowing thoughts (narrow internal)**
   While resting comfortably with your eyes closed, pay particular attention to the thoughts that your mind brings to the surface. This is to be done with a non-judgmental and passive attitude. Passively recognize the thoughts and allow them to come into and leave the mind at their own pace (2 minutes).

4. **Choose a problem (narrow internal)**
   Choose an issue that has been bothering you and ask your mind to give you as many solutions as it can. As the mind presents each solution, place it into a bubble and allow it to slowly float away. Quietly wait for the next solution to appear. This is also accomplished in a non-judgmental fashion (5 minutes).

5. **Study an object (narrow external)**
   Take any small object that can easily be manipulated in your hand (coin, paper clip, ring, etc.) and focus intently on this object. If the mind becomes bored and begins to wander, refocus on the object. Each time you perform this exercise, change the object (5 minutes).

6. **Listen to your own heartbeat (narrow internal)**

   Close your eyes while in a comfortable position and listen to your heartbeat. Attempt to hear nothing but your own heart beating (3 minutes).

7. **Blank mind (narrow internal)**

   Try to think of nothing. No thoughts, think only of blackness. Attempt to control your mind so that it cannot feed you any thoughts (1 minute).

8. **Shifting exercise**

   This is a three-week exercise for 10 minutes each week. For the first week the athletes need to find an interesting book to read, which has no pictures. The athlete should read in a quiet place and focus on comprehension of the material. The second week, they should read the book and listen to the radio at the same time. Again, they do this for 10 minutes and tell someone what they read and what has been playing on the radio. During the third week, they read the book, listen to the radio, and watch television simultaneously for 10 minutes. This is a fun exercise, and it forces the athlete to learn to shift quickly from one thing to another.

Appendix B

1. Positive cue or trigger words repeated over and over in the mind while competing. Have the athletes select a few of these that have special and powerful meaning to them individually. The mind can only focus on one thing at a time. If it is being positive, then it cannot be negative at the same time (the inverse is equally true).

2. Focus on what you want to accomplish. Talk and think about the objective in the short term. For example, as the golfer strands on the tee, he or she should think and focus on a chosen spot on the fairway and ignore the traps, out of bounds, water, etc.

3. Stay in the present. Become immersed or absorbed in what is happening at the present time instead of thinking of the past or the end result (future).

4. Differentiate between practice self-talk and competition self-talk. Many athletes fail to differentiate between self-talk that is helpful in improving skill and self-talk that is essential when actually in the act of performing or competing. "Practice self-talk" is characterized by questioning, introspection, and searching for ways to change. "Competitive self-talk" is in the present and is characterized by strong affirmative statements. Confident competitive self-talk produces a sense of control and reduces doubt or uncertainty (Reardon, 1995, p. 207).

5. Have two athletes face each other. One athlete spreads his or her arms to the sides. The other places his or her hands on the wrists of the first one. The first one is instructed to think first of a negative thought—something that makes them feel sad and depressed. When they have this thought in their head, they are to nod their head. The second one then attempts to pull their hands and arms down. The first one is instructed to resist this lowering of the arms. The positions are reversed so both partners have the opportunity to think negatively. The second part of this exercise is to think a very positive and arousing thought and again attempt to pull the arms down. Reverse the positions. Inevitably, the athlete will be stronger when thinking positively.

CHAPTER 4

Olympic Games and Sport Psychology

SIDÓNIO SERPA

Olympics, Coubertin, and Sport Psychology

By creating the modern Olympic Games, Pierre de Coubertin consequently influenced the evolution of sports. His belief that being active in sports has important implications for the whole person and society inspired him to discuss topics that, years later, would become central subjects for study, research, and applied work in sports training. The series of congresses promoted by Coubertin (Le Havre, France, in 1897; Brussels, Belgium, in 1905; Paris, France, in 1906; and Lausanne, Switzerland, in 1913) gave rise to new debates and perspectives (Coubertin, 1913a). In Le Havre, the close relationship of sports and moral standards was the main topic, the congress of Brussels focused on the technique of physical exercises, and the event that was held in Paris aimed at bringing together artists and sportsmen under the spirit of renascent Olympism.

However, for all those interested in sport psychology, the Congress of Lausanne held the most importance. Indeed, "it was organized to christen a new science, or to

speak in more precise terms, a new branch of a science, by making it more widely known: sports psychology" (Coubertin, 1913a, pp. 19-20). Under the general theme "Psychology and Physiology of Sports," the program included these topics: solitude and companionship; independence and cooperation; initiative and discipline; formation and training of a team; inborn disposition, or special aptitudes to certain forms of exercises; sporting instinct versus the spirit of imitation or the effort of will; and the need of practicing sports related to the wish of social recognition or the pursuit of beauty, health, or bodily power (Muller, 2000). The discussions also focused on sports training as a means of facilitating the development of will, courage, self-confidence, and mental health. Another interesting subject under the current perspectives of the zones of optimal performance (Hanin, 2000) is the state of mind of athletes who are able to break records. Coubertin had already published an article in *Revue Olympic* (Coubertin, 1913b) under the title "La psychologie sportive [Sport psychology]" in order to approach the main topic of the Congress.

Coubertin's interest in sport psychology was already

demonstrated in the article "La psychologie du sport [Sport psychology]" (Coubertin, 1901), included in *Notes sur l'éducation publique* [Notes about Public Education]. It is an essay about the mental aspects of sport, in which he wrote about motivation, volition, and the discussion related to the intrinsic versus extrinsic origin of motivation. He also referred to the interaction between physical exercise and psychological issues, such as character education, the development of intellectual capacities, and the common frontiers between physiology and psychology. In addition, Coubertin discussed the psychological aspects of different types of sport. By classifying sports according to psychological criteria, he intended to emphasize perspectives that differed from the common ones, which took into consideration solely physical aspects such as strength and dexterity. In an article published in the *Revue Olympique*, the founder of the modern Olympic Games also mentioned the need to consider the psychological individuality in any system aiming to develop physical skills (Coubertin, 1909). In fact, this idea was developed again in a presentation at a conference in the International Exhibition of Brussels in 1910, where he argued that the intensity of the effort required in sports emphasizes individual psychological characteristics, and this requires urgent scientific study by psychologists. Moreover, Coubertin states that *will*, *ambition*, and *competition* are three basic elements that define sport, and they should follow the triple direction of psychology, internationalism, and democracy toward the future (*Revue Olympic*, 1910).

The above paragraphs clearly reveal Coubertin's strong belief that psychology—he named it sport psychology—should be studied to understand modern sports and sports performance, and should be used from an educational perspective toward a better adaptation of athletes to the demands of sports. However, he anticipated the difficulties associated with the development of the psychological approach in sports. Indeed, he stated, "Sportsmen react against self-analysis and be analysed by anyone else. Although they tolerate their blood to be examined, they are not used to have their mind studied" (Coubertin, 1913b, p. 20). Furthermore, when commenting on the difficulties of organizing the Congress of Lausanne, where psychology was introduced as a new topic, Coubertin wrote:

This program, if I may say so, had to be defended against the medical profession and, on the other hand, put over convincingly to the philosophers and teachers to win to our cause; and we had at the same time to start to arouse the interest of sportsmen themselves. (Muller, 2000, p. 456)

Although Coubertin was at the very starting point of sport psychology, which he attempted to promote among scientists and sport performers, many decades passed before sport psychology developed specific research and field work regarding the psychological specificities of the Olympic Games. In 1968, Miroslav Vanek, from the former Czechoslovakia, was the first sport psychologist to be included in a national delegation in Mexico at the Olympic Games (Cruz, 1992). Surprisingly, sport psychologists are not yet included in the list of officials' accreditation for the Olympics, although the work of these professionals with Olympic teams and athletes has greatly increased during the last 40 years.

The Olympic Games: A Special Competition

The Olympic Games are undoubtedly a special competition for those who achieve the right to participate. Although the athletes have years of experience from national and international competitions, the Olympic context is quite different and has important implications regarding psychological adaptation (Gould, 2001; Orlick, 2002; Serpa & Rodrigues, 2001). In fact, a complex group of factors interact to increase the subjective meaning of Olympic participation. One of these factors is the worldwide media impact, as this is probably the biggest event on earth. Athletes' performances are publicly evaluated, and their success or failure is watched by millions of spectators. It is also a multicultural event, joining people from different types of sports and from many different societies, thus contributing to a particular environment that is also a source of distractions regarding the task to be performed. On the other hand, there is just one opportunity every four years to participate in this event—and often it is the only one in the athlete's entire career.

Athletes dream about participating in the Olympics for years and work intensively to achieve it. The moment they finally compete in an Olympic event is the culmination of all the training hours and all the competitions along the preparation process. Now they evaluate this period of their lives. Reaching personal goals may be an outstanding positive experience in the athlete's life, while failing those goals often has dramatic psychological consequences. Both tend to have long-term effects on self-image and self-esteem. Moreover, the athlete is aware that what he or she does in the Olympic competition will also have collective, institutional, and political consequences. As a matter of fact, when he or she loses or wins, the team, the coach, the technical staff, and the managers will also be perceived as losers or winners. In many countries, each athletes' federation or sport organization will be rewarded according to its athletes' competitive results. Politicians will take advantage of participants' achievements and will press them to promote a positive image of their country through their successes.

Therefore, the athlete feels like receiving the heritage of the classic Olympic hero. Together with the social and physical contexts of Olympic participation, it becomes a unique personal experience that necessitates specific preparation.

Specific Olympic Constraints

According to many athletes, the Olympics involve specific constraints that are quite different from other international competitions. For example, the traveling preparation is more complex, including all the arrangements regarding official clothes and other materials to take to the Olympic site, and a high degree of pressure also comes with the accompanying social activities, such as meetings with the government representatives, sponsors, and the press. Often, in the final weeks before the departure, athletes who are not accustomed to being pursued by the press are invited for interviews, TV and radio programs, and photo sessions. As for the Olympic site, accomodations present another set of considerations for athletes. The Games involve an extended stay and the conditions can bring about stressors, such as the fact that the athletes can be placed with roommates they've never met, who may take part in other sports. It may happen that while some have already competed and are more relaxed, others are still in preparation mode, trying to stay mentally focused and in good physical shape. Thus, the conflict of living patterns inside the housing

accommodations may negatively affect those waiting for the big day. The psychological atmosphere caused by the results of the athletes who have already performed may also influence the mental state of their roommates. Other characteristics of the special environment are the great variety of food in the Village restaurants and cafeterias that are open 24 hours a day, the computers, the free access to interactive games and fitness rooms, the discos and cultural events, the biggest names of top-level sports at a mere arm's reach, and more.

Olympians have to deal with a number of distractors in the Olympics sites and should learn how to cope with them (Orlick, 2002). Greenleaf, Gould, and Dieffenbach (2001), when studying American athletes, concluded that the most important distractors during the Olympic Games were the media demands, obtaining tickets for the competitions, getting transportation to the trainings and competitions, the family and significant others, the confusion and excitement of the Olympic environment, and participating in the opening ceremony, which demands a lot of mental and physical energy. In terms of favorable influences, the athletes mention their mental skills, a positive attitude toward the Olympic Games, good team cohesion, good social climate inside the Village, efficient support services, a positive coach-athlete relationship, and good specific physical condition. Orlick (2002) reports other main differences within the Olympic context, such as "the sheer volume of people, the size of the crowds, travel time to and from venues, heavy traffic, lots of delays, and reduction in training time" (p. 8). As in other international competitions, many factors can affect performance, including environmental considerations (e.g., the weather); organizational problems (Peiser & Reilly, 2004); and concerns of host country advantage resulting in biased officiating (Balmer, Nevill, & Williams, 2001, 2003) or familiarity with local conditions (Balmer et al., 2001); however, due to the high personal and social meaning of the Games, the psychological impact may be higher than the impact on performance. These major details should be prepared for in advance, in order to avoid disturbing the athletes during the period when they are supposed to be under control and focused on their tasks.

In this regard the Portuguese athletes and coaches who participated in the Sydney Olympic Games were asked about the specific constraints concerning the Games (Krahe & Serpa, 2003; Serpa & Castro, 2006).

According to both groups, the main constraints were: to be watched by millions of spectators, the public expectations as well as the athletes' own expectations, and the physical and social environment of the Games. Moreover, the performance goals set by the sport organizations, competition among teammates to be selected for the Olympic team, and sport policies regarding the Olympic preparation also contributed to an intense emotional general climate. However, only the athletes mentioned that their performance was affected by their own emotions before and during the Games. Additionally, they reported that the personal significance of participating in the Olympics influenced their psychological adaptation. This suggests that the *inner athlete* may be neglected by coaches in favor of a focus on performance, which they perceive as related to their professional competence. Social-emotional training of the coach could facilitate a better understanding of the athlete, and thus, contribute to increasing the quality of the psychological dimension of the preparation process.

The specific psychological adaptation to the Olympic Games depends on the work done in the preparation period for the event. The more detailed and rigorous this psychological preparation process, the higher the probability to achieve the participants' personal goals. However, athletes participating in the Olympics frequently do not follow the same patterns used to achieve the best results in other competitions, or they fail to focus on the relevant cues (Orlick, 2002). Anticipating the characteristics of the Olympic context and preparing to cope with them will be essential for reaching the competitor's potential. Yet, Grandjean, Taylor, and Weiner (2002) studied the women's gymnastics performance in the all-around final in Sydney, when the vault was incorrectly set 5 cm low for a random half of the 36 gymnasts. They observed that although a number of gymnasts failed their vault performance, they were able to succeed in the following rotations. The authors suggested that the concentration skills of elite athletes in a closed-skill sport led them to refocus successfully for the next task.

Mahoney and Avenar (2005) concluded that male gymnasts who succeeded when competing in the final trials for the U.S. Olympic team had different patterns of cognitive and stress coping strategies compared to their opponents who failed to make the U.S. team. On the other hand, Gould, Guinan, Greenleaf, Medbery, and Peterson (1999), when studying athletes and coaches who had participated in the Atlanta Games, concluded that teams that had met or exceeded expectations had different psychological experiences and strategies than those that had not.

Athletes and coaches usually emphasize the importance of properly planning the international competitive activity during the year before the Games (Greenleaf et al., 2001). The increasing number of competitions, including those in the Olympic sites, is highly beneficial in regard to the optimal adaptation of the athletes. Notwithstanding, the same authors also report a trend toward overtraining, which may be related to the athletes' and coaches' anxiety and perception that the quantitative dimension of the training process may lead to the quality of the Olympic results. In fact, the psychological and physical effects of overtraining tend to decrease performance (Kellmann, 2002), a finding that does not correlate with the desired outcomes of this behavior.

The selection procedures for the Olympic team can be a problematic factor as well (Greenleaf et al., 2001). It may happen that athletes are not fully informed about the procedural details and, therefore, uncertainty may become a source of stress. Athletes request that they be informed about clear criteria very early in the preparation phase, to allow them to have the exact information and to establish correct expectations concerning their goals and plans.

The uniqueness of the Olympic media coverage expresses the social movements and ideologies reflected in this outstanding world event (Real & Beeson, 2002), which lends an additional element of pressure on the athletes. To be prepared for this major factor of the Olympic context, athletes are referred to media training and establish a method to integrate the media into their overall preparation for the Games (Greenleaf et al., 2001; Orlick, 2002; Serpa, 2006a; Serpa & Castro, 2006).

Preparing for Olympic Participation

The international literature reports on the type of athletes' demands as well as psychologists' interventions regarding the Olympic participation. As for the trend of the progressive, increasing, and regular consultation of athletes and coaches prior to Olympic participation, Orlick and Partington were among the first researchers who studied this topic (Orlick & Partington, 1988). These authors concluded that the mental preparation in the years prior to the Games was associated with success. They also concluded that the psychological skills identified as related to good performance were different than the skills provided to those who performed poorly. A profile of good consultants, related to concrete and individually adapted strategies, was suggested.

Gould, Eklund, and Jackson (1992) report that the American Olympic wrestlers performed well when they were able to follow their routines, feel their optimal state, have positive expectations, and use their focusing and motivational strategies. The worst performances were related to the lack of confidence and a mental plan, inappropriate feelings, negative thinking, and routine modifications. In addition to this research, Gould, Eklund, and Jackson (1993) concluded that the most used psychological strategies were (1) thought control; blocking negative and reinforcing positive thinking; (2) attentional focus on the goals and immediate tasks; (3) behavioral strategies related to the use of personal routines; and (4) emotional control by means of visualization and arousal regulation.

Many top-level athletes demonstrate high awareness of what is required to prepare for participation in the Olympics. Serpa (2006b) asked Portuguese athletes from several sports about their psychological needs as they neared the 2004 Athens Games. Their answers referred to the development of skills aimed at psychological regulation and optimizing performance, including imagery; stress and anxiety control; self-confidence management; and crisis management in training and competition, which addresses low motivation, burnout, and frustration. Interaction skills with the media was also mentioned, as well as learning how to use previous experiences from Olympic participations and how to benefit from other athletes' experiences. Other answers included factors such as being prepared for the specific Olympic context and accurate planning of psychological strategies. Finally, they mentioned the need for rigor and efficiency regarding the logistic organization and management of the entire Olympic preparation, due to the high psychological impact on the athletes.

In the inquiry mentioned above, the athletes also suggested some procedures to be followed. For example, they would like to have meetings with other athletes, or former athletes, who already had an Olympic experience. Another suggestion concerned organizing workshops to discuss psychological issues related to the Olympics, involving athletes, coaches, and psychologists, as well as learning and training in psychological skills. Receiving brochures and documents about psychological preparation for the Games would be very welcome by the athletes as well. More specifically, some consultant services were requested: psychological skills training and individual psychological coaching along the whole preparation period, psychological support at the Olympic site, and psychological support after the Games.

The coaches of athletes preparing to participate in Athens also responded to the inquiry (Serpa, 2006b). According to them, psychologists working in the Olympic process must be experts in sport psychology, must be accepted by the athletes, and their intervention must be developed along the whole preparation period, eliminating the possibility of starting the work just when the selection process is finished and the Games are near in time. The coaches agreed with the athletes about the need for workshops concerning the specificity of psychological preparation for the Olympics, and they also suggested that the consultants should help the coaches work with their athletes both in the national team and the daily work in the athletes' own clubs. According to the coaches, the sport psychologist's intervention should focus on the athlete-coach-family triangle as well.

To run for the Olympics consists of a long-term process that includes the preparation, the familiarization, the on-site, and the post-performance phases (Gould, 2001; Orlick, 2002). The preparation phase takes place over several years, when athletes establish the Olympic goal, participate in many national and international competitions, compete in trials for a spot on the Olympic team, and specifically prepare for the Games. The familiarization phase, which should begin weeks or months before the Games, aims at discovering specific characteristics of the site, including physical aspects of the Village, the competition sites, and the city, along with social issues particular to the region. The on-site performance phase refers to cognitive, emotional, and behavioral acclimation to the Olympic context. It aims at helping the athletes to stay on plans and strategies that they are used to following and prevents the possibility of changing their personal patterns, which may affect their performance. Finally, the post-performance phase should involve an objective recall of the entire experience, so that its lessons can be applied in the future.

Working with athletes and coaches who are preparing for the Olympics is also an atypical professional experience for psychologists, and it requires both technical and emotional preparation. Haberl and Peterson (2006) stated that being a sport psychologist consultant during the Olympic project is related to specific concerns and challenges, including ethical ones, mostly due to the fact that the practitioner faces uncommon situations as compared to traditional general psychological services. The authors mention examples such as prolonged travel with teams, dealing with the media, team identification, serving multiple teams and/or athletes simultaneously, and practitioner self-care. Thus, the sport psychologists must prepare themselves for this unique situation and carefully plan their intervention along the project. Moreover, being at the Olympic site is an important way to optimize their psychological work (Pennsgaard & Duda, 2002), and in order to be efficient the consultants need to be personally prepared and psychologically attuned to this context. The following paragraphs will discuss topics related to psychological preparation for the Olympics and the related interventions to be done by the sport psychologists.

Interventions Before the Games

Psychological training must be developed in the years before the Games. Introducing new elements, such as mental training, close to or during the Games will demand new adaptation processes and disturb the athlete's emotions and cognitions, consequently adding additional stressors. Therefore, the psychologist must focus on very specific issues that will facilitate the psychological approach to the event and introduce these to the athletes months or weeks prior to the Games.

One of the consultant's most important duties is to advise managers and technical staff regarding organizational procedures and decisions related to Olympic participation. Indeed, logistics and management actions may influence the athletes' mental states and interfere with their performance (Greenleaf et al., 2001; Serpa & Castro, 2006). Athletes often mention that a rigorous and well-organized process leads them to trust in the organization's system and staff. This enhances their confidence and positive expectations. One major topic to be decided is whether the athletes should participate in the Opening Ceremony (Gould, 2001). The technical staff, together with the athletes and team managers, must take into consideration several variables for each competitor, such as level of experience, performance and results expectations, and competition schedules. This decision should be made before leaving home and

must be very clear to athletes, coaches, and staff. It is an emotional issue, which often can give athletes more of a sense of belonging at the Olympic Games, that should not interfere with the athletes' mental states or lead to potential problems caused by an unclear situation.

The characteristics of the Olympic Village and the training and competition sites, as well as the general facilities and transportation, are a new context that will demand a strong adaptation effort by the athletes. In order to prevent an additional source of stress, the athletes must be in contact with this reality as soon as possible. Virtual visits via internet, video, or photos, accompanied by a review of specific coping strategies with the coaches and the psychologists, or among teammates, may reduce uncertainty related to the novelty impact and increase psychological regulation. Meetings with athletes who have already participated in other Olympic Games are usually very successful in terms of vicarious experience for those who will have their first Olympic encounter. A prior visit to the Olympic sites by coaches and psychologists would be advisable, aiming at establishing an efficient psychological training plan.

Being an outstanding worldwide event, the Olympic Games are a potential target for terrorist actions. Thus, the security procedures are very rigorous and are present in the lives of those who are living in such an environment during the Games. One of the consultant's tasks is to prepare the athletes for this situation. The potential risk must be discussed; the related fears and anxiety must be verbalized; and psychological acceptance regarding the security procedures must be developed.

On-Site Interventions

In order to advance his or her on-site intervention, the psychologist must keep in mind these principles:

1. The essential psychological preparation and mental training has already been done.

2. Now the organizational and logistic issues will be the main focus.

3. Familiar strategies must be followed and new procedures should not be introduced.

4. The consultant must be emotionally prepared for the uniqueness of the Olympic context.

5. The consultant should not be obsessed with "doing (or showing) things," but must be

attentive to individual and group dynamics.

6. The consultant should not force his or her presence, but must be ready 24 hours to provide assistance, if needed.

7. The consultant should not behave like a fan, and must be prepared not to be considered as a central actor. He or she is only a member of the staff who most of the time is asked to take the group photo and not to be in the photo.

In order to organize their interventions, sport psychologists should plan some general strategies to be adapted to the specific situations that will develop on site:

– *Follow the program previously prepared.* The athletes should be adapted to the strategies to be used on site, which should be perceived as meaningful, according to the work done along the preparation phase.

–*Suggest that the athletes visit the Olympic areas.* It is very important for the athletes to visit and carefully observe all the Olympic areas as soon as they arrive at the Village. Familiarity with the sites will help personal adaptation, facilitate imagery, and contribute to better displacement planning. The sport psychologist may accompany them if they feel comfortable with this; however, in terms of mental and emotional readiness, it may be helpful to go alone to the competition site to calmly observe it and know it in detail, and to introject this experience.

– *Help performers' exchanges generate a positive atmosphere and facilitate effective solutions.* The psychological pressure during the Olympics may generate some interpersonal tension and conflicts. The psychologist plays an important role in evaluating the social climate, detecting problems, and taking the correct actions to promote cooperation and a positive social climate.

–*Help athletes and coaches avoid exaggerated concentration on competition and sport goals.* Participating in the Olympic Games is a long-term goal that has finally been achieved. Athletes and coaches want this moment to be one of the most important of their lives, and they focus intensely on performance. Coaches also tend to be anxious, which is due to the fact that they do not control the whole situation. Thus, insisting that the athletes always keep focused is an attempt to regulate the athletes' mental state and increase control over their performance.

These attitudes risk generating high anxiety, which, paradoxically, may disturb the athlete's performance.

–*Help the athletes maintain a balance between being focused on the sports goal and experiencing the Olympic adventure.* Being obsessed by the sports goals and results may prevent the athletes from "living" this unique experience, and may generate frustration in the future. The way the athletes recall their Olympic experience will have consequences in terms of future motivation and emotions. Balance between the right concentration level and the experience of the Olympic situation must be promoted.

–*Promote the use of on-site behavioral routines.* Behavioral routines contribute to psychological regulation, but the specificity of the Olympic context often prevents the athletes from carrying out their usual activities. Daily planning will also help the competitors to keep control over themselves and the situation. The sport psychologist may help the athletes organize their behaviors by establishing and providing daily activities and new routines, which should be done according to the specific situation. Previous visits to the Olympic Village and sites or information from different sources will make it possible to anticipate the preparation. On-site, careful observation on the first day at the Olympic Village will allow for good solutions (Orlick, 2002). As usually happens with other officials, the psychologist's arrival before the athletes will increase the efficiency of his or her work.

–*Be ready to provide psychological support to the coaches.* The coaches' psychological influence in the specific Olympic context is a determinant for the athletes' emotional regulation (Jowett & Cockeril, 2003; Orlick, 2002; Serpa & Castro, 2006). Although the coach-athlete relationship is developed in the preparation years, the emotional and stressful characteristics related to the Olympics may also negatively affect the coaches (Gould, 2001) and their behavior regarding the athletes. In these situations the coaches may not feel at ease to speak about their feelings to other people in order to keep their leadership and self-controlled image. The interventions with the coaches, aimed at helping them maintain emotional balance and communicate positively with the athletes, may be found among the sport psychologist's main tasks.

–*Prepare management strategies focused on the interpersonal relationships.* The Olympics promote mixed emotions, because of the combined atmosphere of celebration and constant competitive tension. Athletes and coaches alike are sensitive to events or procedures that directly or indirectly affect them. Every detail must be thought out and prepared for, especially those related to social issues. The consultant's role is multi-layered with four primary aspects.

1. Interpersonal and communication management.

    Although team-building strategies should be developed before the Games in order to enhance team cohesion and harmony, it is equally important to address interpersonal dynamics during the Games, namely, possible conflicts and relationships among athletes who have never met or have had mainly superficial contact (sometimes they do not play the same sport), and who will have to live together in the same accommodations in the Village. On the other hand, it is also important to have a communication structure in order to keep the members of the team in touch with each other in such a dynamic environment. A communication board at the team accommodations or delegation administrative center, regular group meetings, and a mobile network would provide some practical and efficient solutions to these concerns.

2. Free-time management.

    At the Olympic site, athletes will use some time to train, to eat, and to sleep, but many hours will be free. Thus, a compromise is necessary regarding individual daily activities in order to avoid negative consequences and promote positive effects. Being unoccupied may lead to disturbing thoughts and to increased anxiety. On the other hand, there is the risk of trying to take advantage of everything possible, both social and sport events, and to intensively live the Olympic experience, which may disturb the correct focus and consume energy. Rational and planned time management will release the athletes from an exaggerated concentration attitude, will enable them to enjoy the experience, and will prevent chaotic activity that may affect sport performance.

3. Media management.

    Many people consider the Olympic Games as the most important public event in the world, attracting thousands of journalists. This is an inevitable element of the Olympic process, as it is also necessary to promote sport and to overcome outstanding financial and political investments. Therefore, relations with the press and media management should be a factor to be introduced in the psychological training, as well as in organizational tasks, following the principle of cooperating with the media without damaging the athletes' performances. Athletes and coaches should be trained to interact with the journalists, to positively react to their questions, to develop the best attitudes toward the situation, and to give the most appropriate answers with the athlete's best interest in mind. Contact with the media should be organized by the team's staff in terms of time, duration, place, liaison-person, and documents and information to deliver. The athletes must also be prepared and trained to cope with the contents of the current news.

4. Consulting with managers regarding on-site decision making.

    The Olympic context is a very dynamic system, where unexpected and undesired situations may occur at any moment. Crises may also emerge, demanding prompt action by the managers. Most of the decisions involve people and may affect their psychological state. Moreover, the managers themselves are also under great stress, and most of them are not familiar with or trained to deal with human behaviors and emotions. Therefore, the sport psychologist should be considered as a professional resource for helping the staff to take the best decisions.

—Use observation skills and be reactive. The sport psychologist should be a part of the staff prior to the Games and should know the athletes and coaches personally.

This will enable him or her to detect any unusual behavior and to approach each athlete and coach individually. Emotional support or psychological counseling may be needed, as well as intervention at the social context level. It may also be necessary to assist the athletes regarding psychological recovery between competitions. The sport psychologist must be prepared for crisis intervention regarding individual, interpersonal, team, or management in unexpected situations that may occur during the Olympics and may affect sports performance. Both athletes and coaches can experience various emotional and coping processes during the Games (Pensgaard & Duda, 2002). Some individuals, especially the most experienced ones, may attune their regulation strategies according to the situation, but for many athletes and coaches, a professional intervention in the right moment may be a decisive and positive turning point. Moreover, social support is often a major tool for the athletes' psychological adaptation, and the psychologist, like the coach or other significant persons, plays an important role in this regard.

After the Games

The personal Olympic experience does not end when the athletes leave the Village. It will remain forever and will affect the athlete's career and personal life. The consultant should help the athlete to work and elaborate on the inner experience, to learn from what was done over the previous years, to rationally evaluate the whole process, to re-establish day-to-day life, and to set sport goals and objectives. Gould (2001) reported that when working with the U.S. Olympic team for the Nagano Winter Games in 1998, he took considerable time in performance debriefing discussions with the athletes. Jackson, Dover, and Mayocchy (1998b) suggested that an Olympic post-competition support program should be developed.

Many athletes refer to the fact that no deep evaluation or discussion between themselves and their coaches takes places after the Games. Interviews about 18 months after the events with Portuguese athletes who participated in the 2000 Sydney Olympic Games (Krahe & Serpa, 2003), aiming to study their psychological adaptation to the Olympic competition, revealed that none of them had significantly discussed the subject with their coaches, and most of them cried when recalling their experiences. It could be suggested that the psychological meaning and repercussions for athletes and coaches are

obstacles when it comes to speaking about their Olympic experience. When it is a negative experience, they cannot cope with the feelings related to it, and when it is a positive one, it seems that there is no need to rationalize the positive emotions or to discuss what went well.

Sometimes the athletes' self-evaluation is deeply related to their perception of the media evaluation, which may be very unfair and incorrect in regard to what the athletes objectively did, both in the preparation over the years and in the Olympic competition itself. Moreover, personal feelings of happiness or disappointment may be related to the subjective comparison to the other competitors, classified as better or worse in the Olympic competition (Medvec, Madey, & Gilovich, 1995), or to prior expectations (McGraw, Mellers, & Tetlock, 2005). The sport psychologist should help them rationalize the experience according to the variables that only the athletes and technical staff may understand. The effort to improve as a person and as an athlete, the seriousness and commitment to training and competitions, as well as the important personal experience should be emphasized (Orlick, 2002).

Although the athlete may have not accomplished the realistic result he or she was aiming for, if it is clear in his or her mind that all the effort was made in order to reach the potential, then a personal victory took place. Indeed, the athletes control their behaviors and the strategies and tools to perform well, which increases the probability to obtain the desired result. However, they cannot control other situational variables, such as the opponent's capabilities. This concept should be present during the whole preparation and competitive phases, to prevent unrealistic expectations, and to promote well-adjusted mental states, both during the Olympics and afterwards.

Successful athletes need psychological support as well. Life will be different from that moment on, and sometimes they are not prepared for such a change. Moreover, the important personal goals in the project that guided the athlete's life over many years come to an end, and a sense of emptiness may appear. Jackson, Dover, and Mayocchy (1998a), when studying the repercussions of winning gold medals in Australian athletes, reported positive experiences concerning the whole Olympic and winning experience, new opportunities and material gains, recognition and support, learning experiences, and a sense of achievement. However, negative experiences were also mentioned by the gold medalists, such as a disappointing athletic or professional career in spite of the opportunities and expectations after the Olympic success. Other negative experiences included difficulties in coping with the new personal and social situations, lack of rewards, demands upon the athlete regarding the sport and life context, and memories of a stressful situation at the Olympic Games. In another study, Jackson et al. (1998b) concluded that the Olympic champions often experienced motivation losses, negative effects on their further training or preparation, and detrimental changes to mental approach to training and competition. Yet, others developed good coping strategies and had positive reactions. Especially in those countries that are not typically medal winners, this type of consequence may also concern competitors who did not win a gold or any other medal, but who had met the public's expectations. In many cases, the fact that a young athlete performs well in his or her first Olympic participation will greatly increase the public expectations for the next Games. Therefore, special psychological care will be required.

To conclude, the development of sport psychology is very much associated with the Olympic movement and its founder, who understood the role of this science in a better understanding and optimization of sports performance. The Olympic Games have become the most important worldwide sport event, and have promoted a spirit of exceeding personal goals. Nevertheless, the Olympics are also a very unique context, demanding special psychological adaptation. Therefore, psychological strategies and skills should be worked on in the preparation phase, as well as planned and structured during the on-site period. After the Olympic participation, performance debriefing sessions can help the athletes to make a bridge from this intensive experience to their future projects.

References

Balmer, N. J., Nevill, A. M., & Williams, M. (2001). Home advantage in the Winter Olympics (1908-1998). *Journal of Sport Sciences, 19*, 129-139.

Balmer, N. J., Nevill, A. M., & Williams, M. (2003). Modeling home advantage in the Summer Olympic Games. *Journal of Sport Sciences, 21*, 469-478.

Coubertin, P. (1901). La psychologie du sport. In G. Rioux (Ed.), *Pierre de Coubertain, textes choisis – Tome I, Revelation* (pp. 221-230). Zurich: Weidman.

Coubertin, P. (1909). L'Homme et l'animal, Essais de psychologie sportive. In G. Rioux (Ed.), *Pierre de Coubertain, textes choisis – Tome I, Revelation* (pp. 390-392). Zurich: Weidman.

Coubertin, P. (1913a). The Olympic congresses. In N. Muller (Ed.), *Pierre de Coubertain, 1863-1937 – Olympism, selected writings* (pp. 451-452). Lausanne: IOC.

Coubertain, P. (1913b). La psychologie sportive. In G. Rioux (Ed.), *Pierre de Coubertain, textes choisis – Tome I, Revelation* (pp. 427-429). Zurich: Weidman.

Cruz, J. (1992). El asesoramiento y la intervención psicológica en deportistas olimpicos. *Revista de Psicología del Deporte, 2*, 41-46.

Gould, D. (2001). Sport psychology and the Nagano Olympic Games: The case of the U.S. freestyle ski team. In G. Tenenbaum (Ed.), *The practice of sport psychology* (pp. 49-78). Morgantown, WV: Fitness Information Technology.

Gould, D., Eklund, R., & Jackson, S. (1992). 1988 U.S. Olympic wrestling excellence: I. Mental preparation, precompetitive cognition, and affect. *The Sport Psychologist, 6*, 358-382.

Gould, D., Eklund, R., & Jackson, S. (1993). Coping strategies used by U.S. Olympic wrestlers. *Research Quarterly for Exercise and Sport, 1*, 83-92.

Gould, D., Guinan, D., Greenleaf, C., Medbery, R., & Peterson, K. (1999). Factors affecting Olympic performance: Perceptions of athletes and coaches from more and less successful teams. *The Sport Psychologist, 13*, 371-394.

Grandjean, B. D., Taylor, P. A., & Weiner, J. (2002). Confidence, concentration, and competitive performance of elite athletes: A natural experiment in Olympic gymnastics. *Journal of Sport & Exercise Psychology, 24*, 320-327.

Greenleaf, C., Gould, D., & Dieffenbach, K. (2001). Factors influencing Olympic performance: Interviews with Atlanta and Nagano U.S. Olympians. *Journal of Applied Sport Psychology, 13*, 154-184.

Haberl, P., & Peterson, K. (2006). Olympic-size ethical dilemmas: Issues and challenges for sport psychology consultants on the road and at the Olympic Games. *Ethics & Behaviour, 16*, 25-40.

Hanin, Y. L. (2000). Individual zones of optimal functioning (IZOF) model: Emotion-performance relationships in sport. In Y. L. Hanin (Ed.), *Emotions in sport* (pp. 65-90). Champaign, IL: Human Kinetics.

Jackson, S. A., Dover, J., & Mayocchy, L. (1998a). Life after winning gold: I. Experiences of Australian Olympic gold medalists. *The Sport Psychologist, 12*, 119-136.

Jackson, S. A., Dover, J. & Mayocchy, L. (1998b). Life after winning gold: II. Coping with change as an Olympic gold medalist. *The Sport Psychologist, 12*, 137-155.

Jowett, S., & Cockerill, I. M. (2003). Olympic medalists' perspective of the athlete-coach relationship. *Psychology of Sport & Exercise, 4*, 313-331.

Kellmann, M. (2002). Underrecovery and overtraining: Different concepts—Similar impact? In M. Kellmann's (Ed.), *Enhancing recovery—Preventing underperformance in athletes.* (pp. 3-24). Champaign, IL: Human Kinetics.

Krahe, M., & Serpa, S. (2003). Estados psicológicos e o processo de adaptação dos atletas aos Jogos Olímpicos de Sydney 2000: percepção dos atletas. In P. Castro, R. Novo, M. Garrido, R. Pires, & C. Mouro (Eds.), *Proceedings of the V National Symposium of Research in Psychology* (pp. 115-116). Lisbon: Portuguese Association of Psychology.

Mahoney, M. J., & Avenar, M. (2005). Psychology of the elite athlete: An exploratory study. *Cognitive Therapy and Research, 1*, 135-141.

McGraw, A. P., Mellers, B. A., & Tetlock, P. E. (2005). Expectations and emotions of Olympic athletes. *Journal of Experimental Social Psychology, 41,* 438-446.

Medvec, V. H., Madey, S. F., & Gilovich, K. (1995). When less is more: Counterfactual thinking and satisfaction among Olympic medalists. *Journal of Personality and Social Psychology, 69,* 1284-1296.

Muller, N. (Ed.). (2000). *Pierre de Coubertain, 1863-1937 – Olympism, selected writings.* Lausanne: IOC.

Orlick, T. (2002). Excelling in the Olympic context. *Journal of Excellence, 6,* 5-14.

Orlick, T., & Partington, J. (1988). Mental links to excellence. *The Sport Psychologist, 2,* 105-130.

Peiser, B., & Reilly, T. (2004). Environmental factors in the Summer Olympics in historical perspective. *Journal of Sport Sciences, 22,* 981-1002.

Pensgaard, A. M., & Duda, J. (2002). "If we work hard we can do it": A tale from an Olympic (gold) medalist. *Journal of Applied Sport Psychology, 14,* 219-236.

Real, M., & Beeson, D. (2002). New narratives in the Olympic Games: Sport, hegemony, and the public sphere. *Paper presented to the Working Group on Media and Sport, 23rd Conference and General Assembly of the International Association for Media and Communication Research,* Barcelona, Spain, July 21-26.

Revue Olympic (1910). Psychologie, internationalisme, démocratie. In G. Rioux (Ed.), *Pierre de Coubertain, textes choisis – Tome I, Revelation* (pp. 423-426). Zurich: Weidman.

Serpa, S. (2006a). Olympic participation and the coach's role. In F. Boen, B. De Cuyper, & J. Opdenacker (Eds.), *Current research topics in exercise and sport psychology in Europe* (pp. 59-67). Leuven: Lanoo Campus Publisher.

Serpa, S. (2006b, October). *Psychological specificity of Olympic participation.* Paper presented at the International Forum Psychology of Olympic Excellence, Taipei, Taiwan.

Serpa, S., & Castro, T. (2006). Psicología de los Juegos Olimpicos: La percepción de los entrenadores, *Revista de Psicología del Deporte, 15,* 183-189.

Serpa, S., & Rodrigues, J. (2001). High performance sports and the experience of human development. In G. Tenenbaum (Ed.), *The practice of sport psychology* (pp. 101-128). Morgantown, WV: Fitness Information Technology.

CHAPTER 5

Sport Psychology Service Provision at Elite International Competitions

JUDY L. VAN RAALTE AND ALBERT J. PETITPAS

Sport psychologists who create and provide sport psychology programs for elite athletes traveling to international competitions such as the Olympic Games face a daunting task. Pre-event preparation, intervention implementation, and program evaluation are discussed in this chapter, using the service delivery heuristic described by Poczwardowski, Sherman, and Henschen (1998) as a framework. We also provide guidelines for sport psychologists traveling and working with elite competitive athletes and teams.

Preparation

Sport psychology service has roots in both psychology and sports sciences (Vealey, 2007). Thus, sport psychologists who are preparing to work with elite athletes often use approaches that rely on fundamental skills derived from both coaching and counseling or their clinical work (Andersen, Van Raalte, & Brewer, 2001). Flexibility and broad expertise are essential when work-ing in competitive sport environments, as practitioners are often called upon to deliver services addressing a wide range of issues—in unusual locations (e.g., a locker room, a high jump pit) and at unusual times (e.g., right before a major competition, during the middle of the night) (McCann, 2000).

Sport psychology consultants who have had the opportunity to establish relationships and work with teams and athletes well before major competitions are able to use assessments, observations, and interviews to determine the sport psychology needs of the teams and athletes with whom they are working. Elite athletes' re-sponsiveness to this type of sport psychology approach may well be favorable; a survey of elite athletes from various countries indicated that 81% rated mental prepa-ration as being very important (Heishman & Bunker, 1989). The benefits elite athletes derive from mental skills training impacts a number of areas of sport func-tioning and performance. McPherson and Kernoodle (2002) found that elite athletes tend to express less frustration, more confidence, and less desire to quit the sport than do novice athletes.

Having sufficient time to develop rapport enables sport psychology practitioners to understand the needs of teams and athletes and facilitates development of appropriate frameworks for intervention. By recognizing and comprehending the team's unique issues, sport psychologists are better able to identify mental skills areas that might benefit from greater attention and are more likely to take notice of athletes who suffer declines in key areas, such as productive thinking (i.e., the ability to manage thoughts in a manner that leads to well-being and success). These sport psychologists may also anticipate sport psychology issues that could arise on the road and implement programming and interventions to address them prior to major competitive events, before serious problems arise or small lapses develop into major crises (Halliwell, 1989; May & Brown, 1989; McCann, 2000).

There are times, however, when sport psychologists are assigned to work with large teams, athletes who live and/or train in distant locations, or athletes recently added to competitive groups. In these cases, sport psychologists may not have the chance to meet or work closely with everyone involved. Therefore, it is useful for the sport psychology consultant to ensure that all parties have been contacted and are aware of his or her professional philosophy, services provided, and professional boundaries (Van Raalte, 2003).

Making Contact

In advance of international competitions, the sport psychologist should begin discussion with relevant administrators, national governing bodies, coaches, and athletes. These conversations will help determine how sport psychology services fit into the total service delivery system. A number of sport psychology organizations, such as the Association for the Advancement of Sport Psychology and the International Society of Sport Psychology, have begun addressing issues of sport psychology credentialing. At present, however, it is unlikely that sport psychology practitioners will be issued "sport psychology" credentials at the Olympics or other major international competitions. The type of credentials issued can have important ramifications for access to athletes and competition venues. In recent years, sport psychologists have held credentials as coaches, medical doctors, and even horse owners, among others.

Contact with athletes prior to and during international competitions is ideally made in person. However, it is also possible to stay in touch via mail, telephone, and e-mail. It can be convenient to use electronic sources to contact athletes, but it should be noted that these communications are not confidential and can be overheard or intercepted and recorded.

In addition to confidentiality issues, ethical issues have been raised about computer-assisted consulting, particularly with regard to the adequacy and appropriateness of online intervention in the treatment of sensitive issues (Maheu & Gordon, 2000). Coomey and Wilczenski (2005) found that the perception of social-emotional information was significantly affected by the technological modality (i.e., text, audio, video communication) by which it was delivered. Participants in their research indicated that they perceived text-based messages to be more emotionally charged than the same messages presented via audio or video. As athletes are likely to experience social-emotional concerns in the period of time around important competitions, the potential for misinterpretation of e-mail and other electronic communications may pose a challenge to the provision of optimal services. Electronic media may be most useful for scheduling purposes with teams and athletes. A study by Zizzi and Perna (2002) indicated that athletes who were randomly assigned to contact their sport psychology consultant via electronic means (i.e., e-mail, web pages) were more likely to make contact and complete assignments than athletes who were asked to contact their sport psychology consultants via traditional methods (e.g., in-person meetings). Advances in technology present a challenge to the development of ethical policies in sport psychology that can fully address issues pertaining to the appropriate delivery of services via various technology modalities. At present, it may be best to rely upon mobile phones and e-mail primarily for the scheduling of meetings.

Sport psychologists and the athletes they work with will benefit from anticipating and preparing for the challenges arising from media attention, other external sources, team factors, and individual concerns that can develop around major international competitions. For example, media attention is likely to be greater at important international competitions than at other competitive events. Although some athletes enjoy interacting with the media and following media reports of their performances, many find the increased attention overwhelming, or at minimum, distracting. Athletes who can anticipate the surge in media attention and plan a productive strategy to manage it (e.g., setting availability for interviews and spending limited time reading or watching coverage of the games so that it does not interfere with training and rest) are likely to perform better and enjoy their experiences more than athletes who are unprepared (Baillie & Ogilvie, 2002).

Additional pressure may also arise from external sources, such as family members. Family members who do not usually attend competitions may want tickets, and therefore, may be in proximity to the athletes during events such as the Olympics. The presence of family members may provide athletes with additional support. However, being in touch with and/or spending time with family members can affect athletes' competitive routines, leading to a disruption in normal scheduling, preparation, and eating patterns. Clear communication with family members about availability, commitments, and needed support prior to departure can alleviate some of these problems.

Unpredictable scheduling, disrupted routines, and unexpected events are also common at major competitions. Athletes who are able to block distractions out, "let things go," and understand that "this is how it is" or "you get what you get" may be better able to channel their energy into competition goals and are less likely to be angry and frustrated (Jones, 2000).

Although team factors such as coaching decisions, amount of playing time allotted, and team cohesion can be problematic at any time, these concerns can become magnified at important elite competitions. In some cases, team problems begin as soon as the team is selected, especially if the roster is not exactly as expected. In sports where athletes compete in both team and individual events, it can be particularly difficult to develop team cohesion. The impact of effective team-building activities can be quickly reversed following intense individual competition. More experienced athletes can share their knowledge with less experienced athletes about managing the pressure, media demands, transportation challenges, and other issues. These discussions benefit the novices, who tend to underestimate the pressures and often think that international competitions are "no big deal." Experienced athletes know that anything may go wrong and that they must accept the situation and still perform. Veterans of elite competitions often just want to "get through" the experience.

Finally, individual challenges can affect performance. Athletes may suffer from unexpected injuries or become ill. Their desire to excel on the world stage can in some cases contribute to a change in normal routine that leads to poorer performances or other negative outcomes. Being familiar with the medical and psychological resources available during the games can be extremely helpful for those who have a need for additional services and comforting even for athletes who do not encounter individual challenges.

Professional Philosophy

Poczwardowski et al. (1998) highlighted the importance of developing a philosophy of service delivery. This philosophy must be one that is compatible with the realities of international competitions, during which sport psychology work is often practiced in nontraditional meeting places, in limited time, and under pressure (Gould & Roberts, 1989; McCann, 2000). An educational approach focusing on mental skills has been widely used in elite competitive settings (Gipson, McKenzie, & Low, 1989; Halliwell, 1989; McCann, 2000). This type of approach is based on the idea that the provision of information pertaining to mental skills and the provision of assistance in implementing and acquiring skills under increasing competitive pressure will enable athletes to optimize their performance (Vealey, 2007). In some cases, clinical approaches focusing on behaviors and problematic personality processes have been used to help athletes make changes via the provision of remedial therapy (Vealey, 2007). However, clinical interventions are typically used to address specific concerns of individuals. A crisis intervention model may be particularly valuable for work with athletes at elite international competitions.

Crisis intervention models start with four basic assumptions: (1) Responses to significant crises are not pathological, although they may cause athletes to exhibit symptoms associated with mental illness such as denial, anxiety, or depression; (2) these responses are affected by athletes' relationships with significant others such as coaches, teammates, and family members; (3) individual athletes may react to a stressful competitive event in ways that differ from the reactions of other athletes exposed to the same stimuli (e.g., one athlete may become extremely frustrated when a coach reduces her or his playing time, while another athlete may become motivated to perform better); and (4) individual athletes vary in the length of time that they are affected by a particular crisis (Bloom, 1997; Shapiro & Koocher, 1996). Given these basic assumptions, sport psychologists employing crisis intervention models work to provide their athletes with support, to convey optimism, and, if necessary, to make an effort to enhance self-esteem (see also Pedulla & Pedulla, 2001). It is important to note that crisis intervention approaches are effective in the short term, as indicated by a recent meta-analysis (Roberts & Everly, 2006), but are not a panacea. Booster sessions are often necessary for several months or as long as a year after a crisis.

Comprehensive sport psychology services that extend beyond the games themselves and address the long-term needs of elite athletes can be organized in accordance with the guidelines outlined in the Life Development Intervention Model (Danish, Petitpas, & Hale, 1993). This approach begins with the assumption that participation in an elite international competition, like any significant life event, should be considered a process that includes the anticipation, actual occurrence, and aftermath of the event. As such, interventions can take place before, during, and after the event.

Interventions that occur before elite international competitions are considered to be enhancement strategies, and are used to help participants prepare for future events by developing appropriate coping techniques. With the proper mental skills, athletes can prepare for various potential stressors at the Games (e.g., added pressure, family distractions, delays, new routines, and other unexpected events). If anxiety is increased by the unknown or unexpected events, then enhancement strategies can provide athletes with a greater sense of control and predictability that can lower the experienced levels of stress (Danish, Petitpas, & Hale, 1992).

During elite international competitions, support interventions can provide athletes with the various types of assistance that they may need during the games. Because they are away from home, athletes should plan to have individuals available to help them effectively cope with the competition experience, through the provision of practical, emotional, challenging, informational, and technical support . Although national governing bodies may provide some of these support services, athletes will often feel more secure knowing that they have their own resources available.

Comprehensive sport psychology services should also include counseling interventions to help athletes who may require assistance dealing with the aftermath of the games. Athletes who are depressed because they did not meet their expectations or athletes who may have incurred a potentially career-ending injury are just two examples of situations in which individuals would benefit from psychological support services. Comprehensive sport psychology service delivery allows sport psychologists to help athletes prepare for and effectively cope with events they may encounter before, during, and after the games, ranging from the minor (e.g., jet lag) to the major (e.g., athlete suicide) (Buchko, 2005).

Professional Boundaries

All services will be more effective if athletes, coaches, and National Governing Bodies (NGBs) know what to expect from the sport psychologist. Ideally, roles, boundaries, and the specifics of the referral process are clarified and explored during meetings and workshops before the international competition begins.

Individual or small group training meetings are particularly helpful in teaching coaches, athletes, and other professionals how to refer athletes to sport psychology services, and increase the likelihood that athletes will follow through with the referral (Gordin & Henschen, 1989; Murphy & Ferrante, 1989). The training can be brief, informing these professionals that it is effective for them to: (a) tell the athlete that they want to make a referral for sport psychology services, and (b) ask the athlete if they would like to talk with the sport psychology consultant. Once the referral has been made, interested athletes can approach the sport psychologist directly, or the person making the referral can initiate contact. The referral training protects the dignity and privacy of the athletes, and for those making referrals, it builds confidence in their ability to correctly refer athletes (Van Raalte, 2003).

Given the chaotic nature of international competition, it is useful to provide information both verbally and in writing. Baillie and Ogilvie (2002) suggest that sport psychology consultants working with elite teams address a number of key issues in their contracts, including financial terms and professional issues. Financial terms might include level of compensation, terms of payment, time period during which the contract is in effect, and clauses by which either side may prematurely terminate services. Issues such as professional boundaries, specific competencies, and referrals should also be addressed.

Intervention Implementation

Sport psychologists working at elite competitions usually prepare informational materials for athletes and coaches, but often find that these materials are not the primary focus of services provided at international competitions (Peterson, 2001). Given that the needs of each group and individual are different, it can also be useful to conduct assessments prior to interventions and to evaluate programming after competitions.

Assessment

Assessment can include interviews conducted in person, behavioral observation, videotape review, coach reports, and standardized and other questionnaires (McCann, Jowdy, & Van Raalte, 2002). Athletes and coaches often seem willing to complete questionnaires during down time, such as airport layovers or long flights (Baillie & Ogilvie, 2002). Before assessment takes place, it is essential for sport psychologists to inform athletes and coaches with whom (if anyone) the results of the assessments will be shared, and to ensure that appropriate levels of security and confidentiality of the assessments are maintained.

Service Type and Organization

The services provided by the sport psychologist reflect the knowledge and talents of the sport psychologist and the needs of the athletes and coaches (Gipson et al., 1989; Gould & Roberts, 1989; Hardy & Parfitt, 1994; May & Brown, 1989; McCann, 2000; Murphy & Ferrante, 1989; Peterson, 2001). Examples of the services that might be provided include: pre-competition letters on relevant topics (e.g., stress management, concentration, sleep, communication, motivation, anxiety, nutrition/food, teamwork, family relationships), individual and group meetings during competition, assistance with concerns about personal safety and security, and referral to a psychiatrist when needed (Van Raalte, 2003).

Sport psychology consultants who have developed a rapport and a good working relationship with athletes prior to major competitions typically have some understanding of the nature and history of the athletes' performance issues. As a result, they are in the best position to provide brief interventions to athletes who may be having a difficult time adjusting to the pressure of elite competitions, who may not know how to handle all the distractions surrounding an elite event, or who may be struggling with self-doubts or other issues brought on by the newness or importance of a major international competition.

Giges and Petitpas (2000) have coined the phrase *brief contact interventions* to describe the relatively short (i.e., less than 20 minutes in length) interactions that can take place in field settings. These often unplanned interactions between athletes and sport psychologists take advantage of "teachable" moments and typically help athletes gain different perspectives on their present situations. For example, sport psychologists who have ongoing relationships with athletes may pick up on something in their gestures, facial expressions, body language, or words that are out of the norm for that individual. These atypical behaviors provide entry points where sport psychologists can explore these athletes' perceptions of their situation in more depth, and by so doing, assist them in gaining a better understanding of their experiences. Once the content of an entry point is examined in more depth, sport psychologists may be able to initiate small changes in behavior or perceptions that might lead to an interruption in an entire pattern of non-productive thinking or behavior.

Sport psychologists may be called upon to assist athletes with whom they do not have the benefit of a previously established relationship. This type of situation might involve an athlete who has experienced an acute injury while performing or has been confronted with some other type of unexpected trauma. When this is the case, service delivery of crisis intervention is limited, and sport psychologists typically strive to use empathetic listening and emotional support to assist athletes in returning to their pre-crisis state of equilibrium. The goal of crisis intervention is not to address any underlying pathology or difficulty, but to create a supportive and psychologically safe environment where athletes are better able to use their own coping resources.

Program Implementation

Program implementation during international competitions can be extremely challenging due to issues of access, training, schedules, and housing location of the sport psychologist and athletes. Hotel and mobile telephone availability are extremely important to help schedule meetings. Much sport psychology work is done informally outside of the traditional office setting—waiting in lines, at meals, and on busses (McCann, 2000).

Some sport psychologists feel pressure during international competitions to provide sufficient or extra services that give value equal to or even above the amount of money that they have been paid. It is important for sport psychologists to make sure that they provide services as needed, but do not add unnecessarily to the demands on athlete time. Sport psychologists may spend a good part of each day just "hanging out" or interacting informally with coaches and athletes. Although these interactions may not seem like "real" sport psychology service delivery, they are not wasted time. Indeed, Andersen (2000) noted that hanging out with athletes can be a crucial part of relationship development.

Given the possibility that misunderstandings occur and indeed are more likely to take place when people are under the pressure associated with important competitions, it is beneficial for the specific nature of sport psychology services to be clearly defined at the start of consultation and revised over time as personnel and the needs of particular coaches, teams, and athletes change. It is especially important to address issues pertaining to sport psychology consultant availablility as some athletes and coaches prefer to contact a sport psychology consultant only when they desire assistance and other athletes and coaches prefer to have the sport psychology consultant "hanging around" to provide services on the spot when needed. Often informal contact and roles (e.g., messenger, water bottle holder) are adopted by sport psychologists while hanging out. Maintenance of appropriate boundaries in informal circumstances can help prevent dual relationship ethical dilemmas. One beneficial outcome of the delivery of appropriate ethical services is that in many cases, the relationships formed between athletes and sport psychologists during competitions lead to continued services after the event has ended.

Self-Management

At international competitions, sport psychology consultants may be on call 24 hours per day. The emotional work involved in constantly caring for others can be stressful and create a state of *compassion fatigue* (Weiss, 2004). The negative consequences of stress for helping professionals include emotional exhaustion and anxiety, decreased attention and concentration, impaired decision-making skills, disrupted personal relationships, and loneliness (Shapiro, Brown, & Biegel, 2007). Self-awareness, self-regulation or coping, and a balancing of self and others' interests have been shown to be particularly important self-regulatory skills for caregivers (Baker, 2003). In order to offer the best service to athletes during competition, the consultant should have proper rest, exercise, and a balanced diet; maintain social and professional support networks; and manage professional obligations, such as keeping appropriate and secure records.

Unlike people working in other helping professions, it is likely that all sport psychologist behaviors, including "relaxing," can and will be observed by the media and others. Maintaining professional standards even when relaxing is important. Creating a mechanism for supervision and support from colleagues at international competitions or at home can serve as a professional stress reduction and self-management tool that counters life in this "fish bowl" environment (Van Raalte & Andersen, 2002). Although e-mail and mobile telephones are an easy way to contact colleagues and supervisors, issues of confidentiality should be treated with great care.

Program and Sport Psychology Consultant Evaluation

Countless intervention programs are implemented every year. Unfortunately, the effectiveness of these programs has generally remained unknown. Indeed, a review of stress management research indicated that while over 600 articles discussed the importance of stress management programs, only 24 articles reported data pertaining to the evaluation of such programs (Shapiro, Shapiro, & Schwartz, 2000). Evaluation of sport psychology programming is worth the extra investment of time and effort. There is great benefit in allowing sport psychology consultants to identify strengths and shortcomings in their work and to create improved programming that meets the needs of important stakeholders such as coaches and NGBs (Owen, 2006). Reports providing evidence for the effectiveness of programming increases the likelihood that NGBs and coaches will fund sport psychology services in the future. Without evaluation research, conclusions cannot be drawn about the value of interventions and services, and appropriate modifications for future programming are less likely to be made.

To assess the outcome of sport psychology services, it is useful to garner feedback from athletes, coaches, and staff. Positive responses may be used to refine service delivery and to provide evidence of the need for sport psychology services at future competitions. Response rates to post-competition questionnaires can be low. Keeping questionnaires short and/or including them with other official post-competition materials can be helpful in enhancing response rates (Van Raalte, 2003). It is also valuable to conduct a self-assessment to identify strengths and weaknesses of the experience as a whole and to use that information to improve service delivery (Baillie & Ogilvie, 2002). Many sport psychology consultants have adopted variations of the "Good–Better–How?" model of self-evaluation that was first introduced by Nilsson, Marriott, and Sirak (2007) as a post-shot routine strategy for professional golfers. In this format, consultants first identify what they did well, so as to not discount or lose sight of any improvements or skills they displayed. Next, consultants determine what they could have done better or areas in which they could have focused more attention. Finally and most importantly, consultants consider how they could be more effective in the specific situations identified as areas in need of improvement. This approach to self-evaluation typically enables consultants and athletes to avoid and move beyond an exclusive emphasis on errors or omissions, and promotes an emphasis on finding solutions and corrections that lead to self-improvement.

Conclusions

Working with athletes and teams during international competitions is both challenging and rewarding. Advance preparation—involving clarification of the role of the sport psychologist and assessment of team and athlete needs—is essential. Special attention should be paid to maintaining the physical and mental health of the sport psychologist and evaluating the sport psychology program after the international competition. A multifaceted sport psychology program that effectively addresses the needs of the teams and athletes will create a continued and increasing demand for sport psychology services at elite international competitions.

References

Andersen, M. B. (2000). Beginnings: Intakes and the initiation of relationships. In M. B. Andersen (Ed.), *Doing sport psychology: Process and practice* (pp. 3-16) Champaign, IL: Human Kinetics.

Andersen, M. B., Van Raalte, J. L., & Brewer, B. W. (2001). Sport psychology service delivery: Staying ethical while keeping loose. *Professional Psychology: Research and Practice, 32*, 12-18.

Baillie, P. H. F., & Ogilvie, B. C. (2002). Working with elite athletes. In J. L. Van Raalte & B. W. Brewer (Eds.), *Exploring sport and exercise psychology* (2nd ed., pp. 395-415). Washington, DC: American Psychological Association.

Baker, E. K. (2003). *Caring for ourselves: A therapist's guide to personal and professional well-being.* Washington, DC: American Psychological Association.

Bloom, B. L. (1997). The current status of planned short-term psychotherapy. In B. L. Bloom (Ed.), *Planned short-term psychotherapy: A clinical handbook* (pp. 253-269). Needham Heights, MA: Allyn and Bacon.

Buchko, K. J. (2005). Team consultation following an athlete's suicide: A crisis intervention model. *The Sport Psychologist, 19,* 288-302.

Coomey, S. M., & Wilczenski, F. L. (2005). Implications of technology for social and emotional communication. *Journal of Applied School Psychology, 21,* 127-139.

Danish, S. J., Petitpas, A. J., & Hale, B. D. (1992). A developmental-educational intervention model for sport psychology. *The Sport Psychologist, 6,* 403-415.

Danish, S. J., Petitpas, A. J., & Hale, B. D. (1993). Life development intervention for athletes: Life skills through sports. *The Counseling Psychologist, 21,* 352-385.

Giges, B., & Petitpas, A. (2000). Brief contact interventions in sport psychology. *The Sport Psychologist, 14,* 176-187.

Gipson, M., McKenzie, T., & Lowe, S. (1989). The sport psychology program of the USA women's national volleyball team. *The Sport Psychologist, 3,* 330-339.

Gordin, R. D., Jr., & Henschen, K. P. (1989). Preparing the USA women's artistic gymnastics team for the 1988 Olympics: A multimodal approach. *The Sport Psychologist, 3,* 366-373.

Gould, D., & Roberts, G. C. (Eds.). (1989). Delivering sport psychology services to the 1988 Olympic athletes [Special Issue]. *The Sport Psychologist, 3.*

Halliwell, W. (1989). Delivering sport psychology services to the Canadian sailing team at the 1988 Summer Olympic Games. *The Sport Psychologist, 3,* 313-319.

Hardy, L., & Parfitt, G. (1994). The development of a model for the provision of psychological support to a national squad. *The Sport Psychologist, 8,* 126-142.

Heishman, M. R., & Bunker, L. (1989). Use of mental preparation strategies by international elite female lacrosse players from five countries. *The Sport Psychologist, 3,* 14-22.

Jones, T. (2000, September 14). Calmer waters: Bulmer—a veteran in the Olympic battle of nerves. *Calgary Sun,* p. 8.

Maheu, M. M., & Gordon, B. L. (2000). Counseling and therapy on the Internet. *Professional Psychology: Research and Practice, 31,* 484-489.

May, J. R., & Brown, L. (1989). Delivery of psychological services to the U. S. Alpine Ski Team prior to and during the Olympics in Calgary. *The Sport Psychologist, 3,* 320-329.

McCann, S. C. (2000). Doing sport psychology at the really big show. In M. B. Andersen (Ed.), *Doing sport psychology* (pp. 209-222). Champaign, IL: Human Kinetics.

McCann, S. C., Jowdy, D. P., & Van Raalte, J. L. (2002). Assessment in sport and exercise psychology. In J. L. Van Raalte & B. W. Brewer (Eds.), *Exploring sport and exercise psychology* (2nd ed., pp. 395-415). Washington, DC: American Psychological Association.

McPherson, S. L., & Kernoodle, M. W. (2002). Tactics, the neglected attribute of expertise: Problem representations and performance skills in tennis. In J. L. Starkes & K. A. Ericsson (Eds.), *Expert performance in sports: Advances in research on sport expertise* (pp. 137-167). Champaign, IL: Human Kinetics.

Murphy, S. M., & Ferrante, A. P. (1989). Provision of sport psychology services to the U.S. team at the 1988 Summer Olympic Games. *The Sport Psychologist, 3,* 374-385.

Nilsson, P., Marriott, L., & Sirak, R. (2007). *Every shot must have a purpose: How Golf54 can make you a better player.* New York: Gotham.

Owen, J. M. (2006). *Program evaluation: Forms and approaches* (3rd ed.). New York: Guilford Press.

Pedulla, P. M., & Pedulla, M. A. (2001). Sharing the wealth: A model for brief mental health volunteer work in developing countries. *Professional Psychology: Research and Practice, 32,* 402-406.

Peterson, K. M. (2001, Spring). What I did on my summer vacation, or going to "big show" as a sport psychologist. *Exercise and Sport Psychology News, 14,* 7.

Poczwardowski, A., Sherman, C. P., & Henschen, K. P. (1998). A sport psychology service delivery heuristic: Building on theory and practice. *The Sport Psychologist, 12,* 191-207.

Roberts, A. R., & Everly, G. S., Jr. (2006). A meta-analysis of 36 crisis intervention studies. *Brief Treatment and Crisis Intervention, 6,* 10-21.

Shapiro, D. E., & Koocher, G. P. (1996). Goals and practical considerations in outpatient medical crises intervention. *Professional Psychology: Research and Practice, 27,* 109-120.

Shapiro, S. L., Brown, K. W., & Biegel, G. M. (2007). Teaching self-care to caregivers: Effects of mindfulness-based stress reduction on the mental health of therapists in training. *Training and Education in Professional Psychology, 1,* 105-115.

Shapiro, S. L., Shapiro, D. E., & Schwartz, G. E. R. (2000). Stress management in medical education: A review of the literature. *Academic Medicine, 75,* 748–759.

Van Raalte, J. L. (2003). Provision of sport psychology services at an international competition: The XVI Maccabiah Games. *The Sport Psychologist, 17,* 461-470.

Van Raalte, J. L., & Andersen, M. B. (2002). Referral processes in sport psychology. In J. L. Van Raalte & B. W. Brewer (Eds.), *Exploring sport and exercise psychology* (2nd ed., pp. 325-337). Washington, DC: American Psychological Association.

Vealey, R. S. (2007). Mental skills training in sport. In G. Tenenbaum & R. Eklund (Eds.), *Handbook of sport psychology* (3rd ed., pp. 287-309). Hoboken, NJ: Wiley.

Weiss, L. (2004). *Therapist's guide to self-care.* New York: Brunner-Routledge.

Zizzi, S., & Perna, F. (2002). Integrating web pages and e-mail into sport psychology consultations. *The Sport Psychologist, 16,* 416-431.

CHAPTER 6

Free-Throw Shots in Basketball: Physical and Psychological Routines

RONNIE LIDOR

At certain moments during a game, the action stops and a basketball player is suddenly facing teammates and opponents, preparing for what many spectators perceive as an easy shot: the free throw. "Can it be so difficult," ask those who are watching from the stands or sitting on the couch in front of the TV, "to aim the ball at the rim of the basket from a distance of a few meters—when no one is actually interfering—and to throw?" However, when reviewing statistical data on free-throw performance of elite basketball players, it can be concluded that shooting free throws during actual games is not an easy task, but instead is a real challenge for the player, even for those who have reached the highest level of competition. It was reported that the successful free-throw shooting percentages of male college and professional adult players is only about 70-75% (Krause & Hayes, 1994; Lidor et al., submitted for publication). In spite of the advantages associated with shooting free throws, among them the short distance of the shot and the absence of defense, basketball players still have difficulty excelling in shooting from the free-throw line.

While standing on the free-throw line before a shot, the shooter is exposed to a unique psychological situation. He or she is standing alone at center stage, receiving all the attention—from the players on his or her team and those on the opposing team, the coaches, and the audience at large. All eyes are on him or her. At this unique moment, the shooter has to cope individually with a heavy psychological load, particularly during the preparation period prior to the shooting act, without any outside assistance. For example, the shooter must ignore external distractions made by the players from the opposing team (e.g., "trash talk" and hostile verbal behavior) as well as noise generated by the crowd. In addition, the shooter has to cope with internal distracting thoughts that may hinder his or her performance. The shooter might be saying to himself or herself, "I wish somebody else were standing here," "I know I am going to miss the shot," or "I will be out of the game if I miss." He or she has to ignore these distractions, focus solely on the performed task, relax, and aim successfully at the target. This psychological state is not easy to attain under such distracting conditions.

In order to cope with this unique psychological situation, often experienced by basketball players a number of times during the game, players can adopt physical and psychological routines to prepare themselves for each time they stand on the line to make a free-throw shot. These routines, what sport psychologists term *pre-performance routines* or *preparatory routines,* have been found to be an effective psychological technique in helping athletes cope with the psychological load placed on them while performing such sport tasks as the free throw in basketball, the serve in tennis and volleyball, or the putt in golf (Boutcher, 1990; Cohn, 1990; Lidor, 2007). If planned in advance and performed consistently, these routines should help performers stay focused during the act, increase self-confidence, and overcome failure. These routines, which can be considered as an integral part of the sport task (Lidor & Singer, 2003), can help the free-throw shooter attain a higher level of proficiency.

This chapter focuses on the use of preparatory routines by basketball players performing free throws during the game. A fair amount of information can be found in the literature on sport psychology and on basketball dealing with various preparatory routines in free throws. Some of these preparatory routines have been subjected to empirical inquiries (see Lidor, 2004; Wrisberg & Anshel, 1989). Other routines were proposed by applied sport psychologists, coaches, and performers based on their practical experience (e.g., Burke & Brown, 2003; Martin, 2006). In some cases, similarities among the routines can be seen (e.g., dribbling the ball a few times before shooting), while in other cases contradictory routines are offered (e.g., focusing attention on the front area of the rim versus focusing on the back area).

This chapter discusses the components crucial to a successful preparatory routine for free-throw shots in basketball. More specifically, the purpose of this chapter is twofold: first, to review the literature examining the use of free-throw preparatory routines—both physical and psychological—from the perspective of both research findings and anecdotal evidence; second, to suggest a routine that can be used by beginning free-throw shooters or those who have not yet established a routine.

The chapter is comprised of five parts. The first part describes the characteristics of the free-throw task in basketball, particularly from a task classification perspective, as well as the settings in which the shot is performed. The second part defines the term *pre-performance* or *preparatory routine.* The third and fourth parts review the sport psychology and basketball literature on the physical routines and psychological routines used in free-throw performances. The fifth part outlines a number of observations made based on the reviewed literature.

Free-Throw Shots– Characteristics and Settings

A free-throw shot is awarded to the player after a foul was made against him or her, or another rule infraction was committed by one of the players of the opposing team (International Basketball Federation, 2008). A sport task such as the free throw in basketball is classified as a *closed motor skill,* which is performed in a stable and predictable environment (Lidor, 2007; Lidor & Singer, 2003). That is to say, the shooter performing a free-throw shot knows in advance how he or she is going to do it, and under what conditions. The environmental settings are stable (e.g., the distance of the shot from the basket, the angle of the shot, and the height of the basket), and the same style of shooting is used by the player each time he or she stands on the free-throw line.

The free-throw shot is also considered a *self-paced task,* meaning the shooter is able to determine when to initiate the shooting act. According to the international rules of the game (International Basketball Federation, 2008), basketball players have 5 seconds to prepare themselves for the free-throw act, with the exception of the 10-second time period available for those playing in the National Basketball Association (NBA) (Whelton, 1988). When players know in advance how much time is available to them, they can release the ball when they feel comfortable and ready to do so. They can decide not only what to do during this preparation interval, but also how to use the time officially allotted to them, taking into consideration their professional needs and preferences.

The Pre-performance Routine–Definition and Aims

Each time the player performs a free-throw shot, he or she can activate a preparatory or pre-performance routine, because the shot is performed in a stable and predictable setting. More importantly, due to the fact that throwing conditions are fixed and anticipated, the shooter can use task-pertinent routines that are prepared in advance and implemented consistently prior to the shooting act.

A pre-performance routine has been defined as a systematic sequence of physical, emotional, and cognitive behaviors that are demonstrated on a regular basis immediately before the execution of self-paced tasks (Lidor, 2007; Moran, 1996). An effective pre-performance routine encompasses physical patterns of movements, thoughts, and emotions associated with the performed task prior to its execution. The main objective of the pre-performance routine is to optimize the preparatory state and the execution capabilities of the performer (Boutcher, 1990). The routine should help performers appropriately manage the time period before the act provided to them according to the rules of the sporting activity.

There are four specific objectives of task-pertinent pre-performance routines: (a) to help the individual stay focused while performing the self-paced task, (b) to prevent negative thoughts and reflections, (c) to block out external distractions, and (d) to develop a plan of action for the performed task (Cohn, 1990; Lidor & Singer, 2003; Moran, 1996). When these objectives are achieved, performers will feel in control over what they are doing before and during the act.

Research in sport psychology has shown that most skilled performers use a consistent routine before they perform self-paced tasks. Among the sporting tasks that have been studied are the free throw in basketball (Wrisberg & Anshel, 1989), the putt in golf (Crews & Boutcher, 1987), the serve in volleyball (Lidor & Mayan, 2005), and the place kick in rugby (Jackson & Baker, 2001). One of the findings that emerged from studies on preparatory routines in self-paced tasks is that skilled performance is typically associated with the consistent use of a pre-performance routine, which is composed of two main components: the physical and the psychological.

This chapter will focus on the use of physical and psychological routines in free throws in basketball. These routines are discussed, based on selected research findings and anecdotal evidence provided by sport psychologists, coaches, and performers. Physical routines are not always composed solely of physical behaviors, and a number of psychological routines also include physical behaviors. However, the physical routines primarily emphasize the physical behaviors used by shooters in their free-throw performances, while the psychological routines mainly stress mental techniques utilized by the shooters to appropriately cope with the psychological load put on them before and during the shots.

Studies on Physical Routines

Physical routines are those overt behaviors that players demonstrate while standing on the line preparing for the shooting act. This part describes the physical behaviors of the shooter that are performed from the moment the shooter is handed the ball by the referee until the completion of the shot. The physical routines are those performed at the free-throw line within the five- (or ten-) second interval available to the shooter.

Research Findings

For the particular purposes of this chapter, only research findings that are directly related to the physical and psychological routines demonstrated by the players are presented. A conceptualized and detailed review of the literature on observational and experimental studies examining the use of routines in free throws (including the ones presented in this chapter), as well as in other self-paced sport events, can be found in Lidor (2007).

Four studies looking at the sequences of physical routines in free-throw shots are reviewed. Two of the studies used high-speed analysis (Southard & Miracle, 1993; Southard, Miracle, & Landwer, 1989), and therefore, a detailed description of the physical routines performed by the players could be obtained. Another study looked at physical routines demonstrated by adult and youth players (Lidor et al., manuscript submitted for publication), and the fourth analyzed the routines of a number of self-paced tasks, including free-throw shots (Southard & Amos, 1996).

In one high-speed analysis study, 10 female college varsity basketball players performing 10 free throws under two conditions—ritual and nonritual—were observed (Southard et al., 1989). In the ritual condition, the players were given unlimited time and freedom of movement before each of the free throws. In the nonritual condition, the players were not restricted by time, but were told to shoot the ball without using any pattern of movements other than those required to perform the shot. Using high-speed analysis, 10 types of ritual behavior were observed: (a) dribble—bouncing the ball; (b) pause—holding the ball for 1 second or less; (c) hold—holding the ball for more than 1 second; (d) bend knees—flexion and extension at the knee joint; (e) bend waist—flexion and extension at the waist; (f) down—moving the ball down with the arms; (g) up—moving the ball up with the arms; (h) ball in—moving the ball toward body; (i) ball out—moving the ball away from body; and (j) release—releasing the ball for the shot.

In another study using a high-speed analysis, similar physical routines were indicated (Southard & Miracle, 1993). In this study, the effect of the timing of ritual behavior on free-throw shots was examined. Eight different ritual behaviors were observed in eight female college players: (a) dribble—bouncing the basketball; (b) pause—holding the ball still for 1 second or more; (c) dip—ball travels downward as a result of bending knees and/or waist; (d) spin—spinning the ball; (e) up-ball—moving the ball upward with the arms; (f) down-ball—moving the ball downward with the arms; (g) up-to-shoot—bringing the ball to position prior to release toward the goal; and (h) shoot—moving the ball from the shooting position to release. A comparison of these behaviors with those observed in Southard et al.'s (1989) study indicated that the acts of dribble, pause, and up-to-shoot were the most common ritual behaviors associated with free-throw performances.

Lidor et al. (submitted for publication) conducted an observational study to explore the sequence of physical behaviors demonstrated by adult and youth male free-throw shooters in basketball during the actual time available to prepare for the shooting act. Specifically, overt behaviors by the players were recorded from the moment they knew that they were going to perform the shot until they actually threw the ball. The length of this time interval was also measured. For the purpose of this chapter, the data related to the official pre-performance time are reported, namely from the moment that the referee handed the ball to the players until they released the ball. It was found that almost all of the players (99.5%) dribbled the ball before they performed the shot. Forty percent dribbled three times, 20% twice,

16% four times, and 12% five times. In addition, 30% of the players rotated the ball while holding it at the free-throw line. On average, the players used about four seconds to prepare for the shooting act while standing at the free-throw line.

In an attempt to determine if preparatory routines display a consistent rhythm across different self-paced activities (e.g., the free throw in basketball), Southard and Amos (1996) outlined eight physical routines performed before free-throw shots by seven male athletes: (a) dribble; (b) pause—no movement for 1 second or more; (c) dip—bend the knees and/or waist; (d) up-ball—moving the ball upward with the arms; (e) spin; (f) up-to-shoot—bringing the ball to an initial shooting position; and (g) shoot—throwing the ball at the basket.

Based on the reviewed studies, it can be observed that the following physical routines are frequently used among free-throw shooters: dribbling the ball a number of times, holding the ball, spinning the ball while holding it, and releasing the ball.

Applied and Anecdotal Perspectives

Physical routines were not only observed in research settings but were also developed and proposed by applied sport psychologists, coaches, and instructors who worked extensively with elite basketball players at both the collegiate and professional levels. For example, one physical routine was jointly proposed by an applied sport psychologist and a well-known college basketball coach (Burke & Brown, 2003). Their routine consists of six steps; two are used before the referee gives the ball to the shooter and four after the player receives the ball. The steps are as follows: (a) getting positioned at the line; (b) waiting for the ball; (c) receiving the ball and dribbling; (d) taking a deep breath while holding the ball; (e) staring at the rim and shooting; and (f) maintaining the follow-through.

Larry Bird, the basketball legend and an NBA coach, advised players to follow a 6-step routine when readying themselves for a free-throw shot (Bird, 1986). Each time the player is awarded a free-throw shot, he or she should (a) get ready—feeling relaxed and confident when going to the line; (b) get set—being in balance at the line; (c) aim—concentrate on the target; (d) fire—release the ball; (e) follow through—the hand should follow the ball to the basket and the eyes should follow the ball until it hits the target; and (f) follow the shot—sense the shot and its outcome.

Joe Whelton, a European basketball coach, argued that foul shooting involves repetition and rhythm; that is, performing the same acts every time and reaching a comfortable fluid motion with the shot (Whelton, 1988). He developed a 5-step routine: (a) anticipation—getting ready from the moment the foul shot is called; (b) balance—stepping up to the line while holding the ball; (c) finding the spot—aiming at the front area of the rim; (d) release; and (e) follow through—maintaining the eyes at the rim until the ball touches the rim.

According to Hal Wissel, an American coach who had experience in coaching basketball at the collegiate and professional levels, the physical routine should include performing a set number of dribbles, checking the mechanics of the shot, using visualization to mentally practice the free throw just before releasing the ball, and taking a deep breath to relax (Wissel, 1994). He emphasized the use of anchor words, such as *yes, net, in,* and *through* while visualizing oneself at the shooting line.

Finally, Tom Amberry, who made 2,750 consecutive successful free throws, performed a routine that is comprised of seven steps: (a) feet square to the line; (b) bouncing the ball three times with the inflation hole up; (c) thumb in channel, third finger pointing at the inflation hole; (d) elbow in; (e) knees bent; (f) eyes on the target; and (g) shooting the ball and follow through (Amberry, 1996).

In general, the physical routines suggested by these practitioners had similarities to those observed in the reviewed studies. Among the main physical behaviors demonstrated by the shooters were getting a position on the line, dribbling, holding the ball, releasing the ball, and following through. The practitioners, however, stressed the importance of the follow-through act performed after the release of the ball, so that the shooter could see the outcome of the shot and react accordingly.

Studies on Psychological Routines

Two psychological routines associated with free throws in basketball are reviewed in the literature: imagery and the Five-Step Approach. The reason for reviewing selected studies focusing on these two particular techniques is that imagery is one of the most popular interventional techniques used in applied sport psychology in general (Callow & Hardy, 2005), and in self-paced sport skills, such as the free throw, in particular (Lidor,

2007). In the Five-Step Approach, this technique was specifically developed to enhance performance of self-paced skills, and therefore it can be applied instinctively when the shooter prepares himself or herself for the shot (Singer, 2002). In addition, psychological routines developed intuitively by practitioners are presented.

Research Findings

Three imagery studies and two Five-Step Approach studies are described.

Imagery

In the imagery studies the technique was examined in two ways: it was compared to other psychological interventions given to the players who took part in the studies (e.g., Wrisberg & Anshel, 1989) or presented in combination with another preparatory technique (i.e., a physical routine) and compared to other interventional techniques (Predebon & Docker, 1992).

One study examined the effectiveness of the visuo-motor behavior rehearsal (VMBR) on free-throw performances in intercollegiate female basketball players (Hall & Erffmeyer, 1983). The VMBR was composed of (a) an initial relaxation phase, (b) visualizing performance during a specific stressful situation, and (c) performing the skill during a simulated stressful situation. It was reported that the players who practiced the VMBR during 10 sessions improved their shooting accuracy.

Another study examined the use of three cognitive strategies—imagery, arousal adjustment, and imagery combined with arousal adjustment—in free-throw shooting performances of 10- to 12-year-old boys (Wrisberg & Anshel, 1989). The cognitive strategies players were compared to the no-strategy players (a control condition). It was found that the players who used imagery combined with arousal adjustment performed more accurately than both the no-strategy players and the players who were taught imagery or arousal adjustment.

Support for the use of imagery combined with another technique was found in another study in which experienced male basketball players were assigned to three training groups: routine (looking at the basket, dribbling the ball a few times, and shooting the ball); imagery/physical (imagining the shot sequence first without the ball, and then while bouncing the ball); and no-routine (aiming at the basket without performing a pre-shot routine) (Predebon & Docker, 1992). It was found that the imagery/physical group outperformed the routine group, which in turn performed better than the no-routine group.

Imagery appears to be one of most popular psychological routines used by basketball players while standing on the free throw line preparing for the shooting act. Either performed by itself or in combination with another preparatory routine, this technique was found in the above studies to enhance accuracy in free-throw shots.

Five-Step Approach

The Five-Step Approach (5-SA) is a strategy that contains five steps: readying (get comfortable physically and attain an optimal mental-emotional state); imagining (briefly mentally picture performing the act as to how it should be done); focusing attention (concentrate intensely on one relevant external feature of the situation); executing (do it; do not think of anything about the act itself or the possible outcome); and evaluating (use available feedback information from which to learn) (Lidor, 2007; Singer, 2002). The five substrategies included in the 5-SA were found to be beneficial for achievement across different self-paced motor tasks. For a review of laboratory and field studies examining the effectiveness of the 5-SA on various sport tasks, see Lidor and Singer (2005).

Two studies examined the effectiveness of the 5-SA on free-throw performances in beginning basketball players (Lidor, 2004; Lidor, Arnon, & Bronstein, 1999). In the first study (Lidor et al., 1999), 13-year-old female and male players participated in six strategy sessions in which the principles of the strategy were practiced. After listening to the strategy instructions, the players performed 15 free throws in each session. Two more retention sessions were undertaken: 15 throws were performed in each of these sessions; however, no new strategy directions were presented. A control group performed an equal number of throws without being exposed to the strategy instructions. The combined data analyses for the boys and girls indicated that the 5-SA players performed with greater accuracy compared to the control players.

In the second study, beginning junior-high female basketball players were taught three strategies—5-SA, awareness, and nonawareness—while acquiring the fundamentals of the free-throw shot (Lidor, 2004). The awareness strategy players were taught to feel their movements before and during the shooting act, to pay attention to small details related to their throw, and to think about what they were doing. The nonawareness strategy players were instructed to plan their shooting act in advance, to focus on one specific cue related to the throwing act, and to let their movements flow. The strategy groups were compared to a control group that practiced the free-throw skill but was not provided with strategy guidelines. It was found that the 5-SA and the nonawareness players performed more accurately than the awareness and control players. In addition, the strategy players increased their preparation time compared with the control players. The 5-SA and the nonawareness strategies, both of which stressed planning the act in advance and focusing attention at one specific cue related to the performance environment, were found to be the most effective routines in free-throw performances.

Applied and Anecdotal Perspectives

A number of applied sport psychologists have established psychological routines based not only on the findings that emerged from empirical inquiries but also based on their long years of experience working with elite basketball players. For example, Brennan (1993) established a psychological routine similar to the principles of the 5-SA (Lidor & Singer, 2005). According to Brennan, the free-throw shooter should develop a centering cue (i.e., the athlete cues himself or herself to an object, a part of the body, or some ritual to direct his or her attention away from distracting events) and maintain a ritual. More specifically, the entire ritual is composed of (a) receiving the ball from the referee; (b) utilizing a centering cue; (c) readying for the free throw; (d) imagining shooting the ball; (e) focusing attention only on the basket; and (f) evaluating the feeling and results of the free throw.

Burke and Brown (2003) proposed not only a physical routine for the free throw, as described earlier, but also a mental routine combining imagery, self-talk, and focusing attention. The routine is composed of six steps; the first two are done before the referee hands the ball to the player, and the next four after the player receives the ball from the referee. In this ritual the player thinks of selected words such as *relax* and *rim* to maintain an appropriate mental state while preparing for the shooting act. The six steps are as follows: (a) using quick imagery and/or thinking *rim* or *hole*; (b) thinking *relax* or *calm*; (c) counting each dribble performed before the shot; (d) thinking *relax* or *calm*; (e) thinking *rim* or *hole*; and (f) thinking *through* or *form*.

According to Mikes (1987), a shooter should have "proper visual awareness, loose muscles, and a rhythmic motion" (p. 74) to accomplish the free throw. He proposed a 6-phase routine: (a) loosening up before stepping to the line; (b) practicing body rehearsal/mental rehearsal at the line; (c) getting comfortable while taking the ball from the referee; (d) focusing at the center of the basket; (e) visualizing success just before shooting; and (f) shooting the ball.

Psychological routines have also been developed by coaches and by performers who achieved excellence in free-throws performances. For example, a 3-phase approach titled The Three "Cs" was proposed by Krause and Hayes (1994), two leading American coaches. Their routine is composed of (a) concentration—focusing on the proper mental approach; (b) cotton—developing a proper mental image (i.e., saying the word *net* before every shot); and (c) confidence—developing respect: remembering a successful shot or analyzing and forgetting a missed attempt.

Another psychological routine was established by Ted St. Martin, who holds the current world record for successful consecutive free throws with 5,221 (St. Martin, 2006). His free-throw routine is composed of a set of physical elements that should be performed in each throw, among them, basic position, grip, release, and follow-through. However, he stressed the necessity of one particular psychological routine—focusing attention. More specifically, the shooter should focus at the back of the rim. This piece of advice is the opposite of the popular instructional tip that coaches usually provide to their players, namely that the free-throw shooter should aim at the front of the rim. According to St. Martin's view, when the shooter is looking at the back of the rim, he or she is actually looking inside the basket, and the target seems even bigger to them.

In the selected review of the most-recommended research and applied literature, the psychological routines described include: imagining while standing at the free-throw line, focusing attention at the front area of the rim, and self-talking while holding the ball.

Developing a Routine for the Free-Throw Shot

Based on the research findings, the applied perspectives, and the anecdotal evidence presented in this chapter, five observations can be made:

First, a number of physical and psychological routines have been proposed in the literature to help basketball players prepare for the free-throw act. However, one fixed routine composed of the same set of physical and psychological behaviors that are used in the same order by all shooters cannot be found. That is, various physical and psychological routines have been proposed for the use of players when standing on the free-throw line and aiming at the rim.

Second, although different shooters use different free-throw routines, a number of physical and psychological behaviors were found to be common among the shooters. These behaviors may not have been performed similarly or in the same order, or have been included in all the proposed routines, but they did appear in the majority of the physical and psychological preparatory routines.

Third, the physical routines that were most shared by the shooters include: getting a position on the free-throw line, dribbling the ball, holding the ball, spinning the ball, releasing the ball, and following through. These routines should be used by shooters when they are developing a physical routine for their own use.

Fourth, the psychological routines most shared by the shooters were: imagining oneself performing the shot while standing on the line, focusing attention on the front area of the rim, self-talking while holding the ball, and evaluating the shot, time permitting. These routines should be included in any psychological routine developed by the free-throw shooter.

Fifth, free-throw shooters should establish preparatory routines according to their own preferences. For beginning shooters or those who have not yet developed a routine, in order to develop the appropriate routine it is beneficial to observe what other shooters do during the five- (or ten-) second interval of preparation before each free-throw shot. Figure 1 presents the main physical and psychological practices that players should consider in their attempt to establish an effective routine. These physical and psychological routines are strongly recommended; however, they should be adopted according to the needs of each specific shooter.

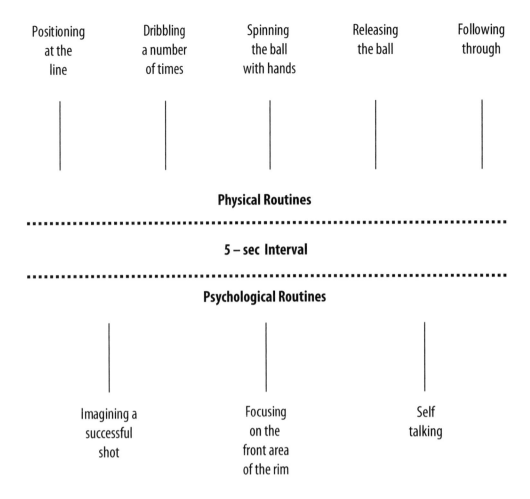

| Positioning at the line | Dribbling a number of times | Spinning the ball with hands | Releasing the ball | Following through |

Physical Routines

···

5 – sec Interval

···

Psychological Routines

| Imagining a successful shot | Focusing on the front area of the rim | Self talking |

Figure 1. Physical and psychological routines in free throws.

References

Amberry, T. (1996). *Free throw—7 steps to success at the free throw line*. New York: Harper Perennial.

Bird, L. (1986). *Bird on basketball*. Reading, MA: Addison-Wesley.

Brennan, S. J. (1993). *The mental edge—Basketball peak performance workbook*. Omaha, NE: Peak Performance.

Boutcher, S. H. (1990). The role of performance routines in sport. In J. G. Jones & L. Hardy (Eds.), *Stress and performance in sport* (pp. 221-245). New York: Wiley.

Burke, K., & Brown, D. (2003). *Sport psychology library: Basketball*. Morgantown, WV: Fitness Information Technology.

Callow, N., & Hardy, L. (2005). A critical analysis of applied imagery research. In R. Lidor & K. P. Henschen (Eds.), *The psychology of team sports* (pp. 37-58). Morgantown, WV: Fitness Information Technology.

Cohn, P. J. (1990). Pre-performance routines in sport: Theoretical support and practical implications. *The Sport Psychologist, 4*, 301-312.

Crews, D. J., & Boutcher, S. H. (1987). An exploratory observational behavior analysis of professional golfers during competition. *Journal of Sport Behavior, 9*, 51-58.

Hall, E. G., & Erffmeyer, E. S. (1983). The effect of visuo-motor behavior rehearsal with videotaped modeling on free throw accuracy of intercollegiate female basketball players. *Journal of Sport Psychology, 5*, 343-346.

International Basketball Federation (2008). *FIBA activities*. Retrieved February 20, 2008, from http://www.FIBA.com.

Jackson, R. C., & Baker, J. S. (2001). Routines, rituals, and rugby: Case study of a world class goal kicker. *The Sport Psychologist, 15*, 48-65.

Krause, J., & Hayes, D. (1994). Score on the throw. In J. Krause (Ed.), *Coaching basketball* (pp. 138-141). Indianapolis, IN: Masters Press.

Lidor, R. (2004). Developing metacognitive behavior in physical education classes: The use of task-pertinent learning strategies. *Physical Education and Sport Pedagogy, 1*, 55-71.

Lidor, R. (2007). Preparatory routines in self-paced events: Do they benefit the skilled athletes? Can they help the beginners? In G. Tenenbaum & R. C. Eklund (Eds.), *Handbook of sport psychology* (3rd ed., pp. 445-465). New York: Wiley.

Lidor, R., Arnon, M., Aloni, N., Yitzak, S., Mayan, G., & Afek, A. (manuscript submitted for publication). Pre-preparatory and preparatory routines in free-throw shots in basketball: How much time is available for the shooters, and what do they do during this time?

Lidor, R., Arnon, M., & Bronstein, A. (1999). The effectiveness of a learning (cognitive) strategy on free-throw performances in basketball. *Applied Research in Coaching and Athletics Annual, 14,* 59-72.

Lidor, R., & Mayan, Z. (2005). Can beginning learners benefit from pre-performance routines when serving in volleyball? *The Sport Psychologist, 19,* 343-362.

Lidor, R., & Singer, R. N. (2003). Preperformance routines in self-paced tasks: Developmental and educational considerations. In R. Lidor & K. P. Henschen (Eds.), *The psychology of team sports* (pp. 69-98). Morgantown, WV: Fitness Information Technology.

Lidor, R., & Singer, R. N. (2005). Learning strategies in motor skill acquisition: From the laboratory to the field. In D. Hackfort, J. Duda, & R. Lidor (Eds.), *Handbook of research in applied sport and exercise psychology: International perspectives* (pp. 109-126). Morgantown, WV: Fitness Information Technology.

Mikes, J. (1987). *Basketball fundamentals—A complete mental training guide.* Champaign, IL: Leisure Press.

Moran, A. P. (1996). *The psychology of concentration in sport performers: A cognitive analysis.* East Sussex, UK: Psychology Press.

Predebon, J., & Docker, S. B. (1992). Free-throw shooting performances as a function of pre-shot routines. *Perceptual and Motor Skills, 75,* 162-172.

Singer, R. N. (2002). Preperformance state, routines, and automaticity: What does it take to realize expertise in self-paced events? *Journal of Sport and Exercise Psychology, 24,* 359-375.

Southard, D., & Amos, B. (1996). Rhythmicity and performance ritual: Stabilizing a flexible system. *Research Quarterly for Exercise and Sport, 3,* 288-296.

Southard, D., & Miracle, A. (1993). Rhythmicity, ritual, and motor performance: A study of free throw shooting in basketball. *Research Quarterly for Exercise and Sport, 3,* 284-290.

Southard, D., Miracle, A., & Landwer, G. (1989). Ritual and free-throw shooting in basketball. *Journal of Sports Sciences, 7,* 163-173.

St. Martin, T. (2006). *The art of shooting baskets* (2nd ed.). New York: McGraw-Hill.

Whelton, J. (1988). *Step by step—Basketball skills.* London: Hamlyn.

Wissel, H. (1994). *Basketball—Steps to success.* Champaign, IL: Human Kinetics.

Wrisberg, C. A., & Anshel, M. H. (1989). The effect of cognitive strategies on free throw shooting performance of young athletes. *The Sport Psychologist, 3,* 95-104.

CHAPTER 7

Talent Development in Sport: The Perspective of Career Transitions

NATALIA STAMBULOVA

"In ancient times, a *talent* represented a fortune that measured the equivalent of approximately 14 kilograms of pieces of silver. Today talent represents our most valuable human asset. It cannot simply be purchased; it is a basis of fantastic careers, of power and fame, but also in many cases of pain, sadness, and misery" (Maes, 2004, p. 117). This chapter deals with talent development in sport, emphasizing its career context (i.e., stages and transitions athletes go through during their multi-year sport participation).

Talent development in sport is a complex and controversial topic. It is naive to think that simply having talent is a guarantee of athletic success. Gifted athletes might feel resourceful and confident early in their careers, but can experience certain barriers when they make a transition to the more advanced levels in sport. As one coach pointed out, "A lot of former world junior champions do not stay in sport. They do not make it or they stay in the sport but they do not seem to go on to greater things.... We...push them too hard too soon

and basically burn them out" (Martindale, Collins, & Abraham, 2007, p. 193).

The course of an athletic career—successful or not—is determined through a complex interplay between genetic, personal, and environmental factors. This chapter focuses on personal (e.g., perceived career demands and coping resources) and environmental (e.g., coaches, parents, sport system, psychological services) determinants of talent development in sport, and advocates a *holistic view of an athlete* and a *holistic lifespan perspective* in helping athletes reach their self-actualization.

Athletic Talent and Career Development

The *Encyclopedia of Applied Psychology* defines talent as specific abilities in applied areas like mathematics, music, sport, or arts (Feldhusen, 2004). This very broad definition is useful, but it does not capture any nuances in such a complicated phenomenon as athletic talent. Sports people use three related but different perspectives—biological, psychological, and social—in understanding athletic talent.

According to the first or *biological* perspective, talent refers to an athlete's innate potential or giftedness (e.g., anthropometric data, structure of muscles, and sensitivity of sensory systems), which is supposed to facilitate the processes of learning and mastering particular sport event(s). Coaches who adopt this perspective often see athletic talent as something magical, which athletes either have or do not have. Naturally, these coaches advocate talent detection and selection based on the following philosophy: Gifted young athletes must first be identified. Then they should be segregated to special groups and provided with the best possible conditions for training, competition preparation, and recovery. This is how a sport system ensures good reserves for elite sports.

The second or *psychological* perspective views talent as the athlete's acquired abilities, competencies, and skills that facilitate athletic performance and help achieve athletic excellence in the chosen sport(s). Coaches with this perspective tend to develop conditions for successful development of all athletes who come to a particular sport and demonstrate a high motivation to succeed. Their professional philosophy can be briefly summarized as follows: Each athlete has unique innate potential. However, this potential is less important for athletic excellence than the athlete's motivation to participate in a particular sport and to continuously work and learn. If a sport system provides good conditions for the development of all young athletes, the best of them naturally build up reserves for elite sports.

These two perspectives clearly reflect the *nature versus nurture* talent debate in sport sciences. Analyzing this debate, Durand-Bush and Salmela (2001) note that in the 1970s-1980s, the major focus of the field of talent development was on the athlete's innate preconditions (the biological perspective) and the development of sport orientation programs, talent selection systems, and sport talent detection models. However, in the 1990s there was a shift toward prioritizing the acquired part of talent (the psychological perspective) and the evolution of talent development and athletic career models. More recently, the latter tendency has been further reflected in talent development environment models (Henriksen, Roessler, & Stambulova, 2007; Martindale et al., 2007).

Finally, it should be acknowledged that the word talent is often used in sport to refer to a *young prospect*. This can be viewed as the third or *social* perspective in understanding athletic talent, because it implies social evaluation and comparison between athletes. Coaches, parents, and managers use normative, comparative, personal, and intuitive criteria to identify this group of young athletes. Being included in this group implies advantages, such as ease of obtaining support and funding; and disadvantages, such as high pressure to meet the achievement standards developed by others.

This chapter makes an attempt to establish a link between talent development and career development in sport. *Athletic talent development* mainly deals with the development of sport-specific competencies and skills, as well as certain performance and athletic excellence issues. *Athletic career development* incorporates talent development with additional, important aspects, such as balancing practice, competitions, and recovery; balancing sport and other activities; interpersonal relationships and social interactions; rehabilitation after injuries, etc. In other words, career development can be seen as a broader context for talent development, where the talent development process builds up the athlete's internal resources to cope with ever-changing career demands.

Each athlete has a unique genetic makeup, personality characteristics and tendencies, compensation mechanisms, and relationships with his or her environment. In their athletic careers, athletes self-actualize through performance enhancement; physical, psychological, and social development; interactions with environment; solving tasks and problems; coping with career transitions, etc. The athlete's ability to develop and effectively use these resources to match the ever-growing demands of an athletic career can be seen as an important part of athletic talent (Hanin & Stambulova, 2004). A summary of athletes' perceived career demands and coping resources, based on the author's multi-year study of Russian athletes (Stambulova, 1994, 1995, 1999, 2000) is presented in the next section.

Career Transitions as Turning Phases in Career Development

Athletic career is a term for a multi-year sport activity voluntarily chosen by the person and aimed at achieving his or her individual peak in athletic performance in one or several sport events (Alfermann & Stambulova,

2007). Descriptive models of an athletic career (see Bloom, 1985; Côté, 1999; Côté, Baker, & Abernethy, 2007; Salmela, 1994; Stambulova, 1994; Wylleman & Lavallee, 2004) define it as a succession of the following stages: the preparatory/sampling stage, the initiation stage, the development/specialization stage, the perfection/mastery/investment stage, the maintenance/final stage, and the discontinuation of competitive sport involvement stage. Career development implies proceeding through all or some of these stages and transitions.

Athletic career transitions can be normative (likely to be experienced by the majority of athletes and therefore predictable by descriptive career models) and nonnormative (less predictable). Each transition phase comes with a set of demands that the athlete has to cope with in order to continue successfully in sport or adjust to the post-career period (Alfermann & Stambulova, 2007).

The study of career transitions of Russian athletes presented below was based on the analytical athletic career model (Stambulova, 1994). The model was initially created based on a comparison of four different approaches found in the Russian psychological and sport science literature that divided a career into a number of stages. A certain amount of overlap between these approaches was taken into account, and the seven normative transitions of an elite athletic career were predicted: the beginning of sport specialization, the transition to more intensive training in a chosen sport, the transition to high achievement sport, the transition from junior to senior sport, the transition from amateur to professional sport, the transition from the peak to the final stage of the career, and athletic retirement. The research aimed at testing this model consisted of three parts, and emphasized specific sets of demands related to each normative transition and the athletes' perceived resources to cope with these demands.

The first part of the study involved qualitative analyses of 552 athletes' written essays titled, "My athletic career." These essays were collected and processed over the course of four years. The participants were student-athletes who were asked to write the essays as an assignment for a sport psychology course at the St. Petersburg State University of Physical Education and Sport. This athletic population represented almost all Olympic sports, different levels in sport (from regional to international and professional), and both genders. The participants were familiarized with the analytical career description model and used it as a framework for

the essay. While some of them were still active in sport at the time of writing, a few had already retired. Therefore, they all used a retrospective approach when writing about the earlier stages and transitions in their career, but for the later stages and transitions, retrospective and actual approaches were employed.

The second part of the study included semi-structured interviews with 16 elite Russian athletes representing both individual and team sports, who had either terminated their careers 1-5 years prior to the interview or were still active as professional athletes. The analytical model served as a basis for the interview guide. The data from the essays and the interviews were analyzed inductively. The aim of the inductive analysis was to identify the low- and high-order themes describing the athletes' perceived demands and resources during each of the transitions predicted by the analytical model.

In the third part of the study, 101 statements that reflected the themes found in the inductive analyses were extracted from the essays and interviews, and combined in the survey titled, "Athletic career transitions" (Stambulova, 1995). A different group of 90 athletes, representing different types/levels in sport and both genders, were invited to express their agreement or disagreement with these statements in relation to their own career transitions. High or very high level of agreement was obtained for 52 statements/themes, which were used for the description of athletic career transitions presented below. Overall, the study provided clear support for *six normative transitions,* because the transitions to high achievement sport and to senior sport were found to greatly overlap.

The Beginning of Sport Specialization

In Russian sport culture, young athletes enter this transition when they come to a specialized sport group (soccer, gymnastics, swimming, etc.) and start to practice under the guidance of a professional coach. It is difficult to determine the clear age markers for this transition because of the range of sport events and gender and individual differences. According to this study, it usually happens between 6 and 12 years old. Before starting to specialize in a particular sport, many athletes would already have tried various types of physical activity within the kindergarten/school physical education classes or in free play with peers. During the first 1-2 years of sport specialization, young athletes typically train 2-3 times per week and begin to take part in competitions by the end of the first year. In the essay and interview data, athletes described the essence of this transition as an adjustment—to sport in general and to the requirements of the chosen sport in particular—to ensure that they made the right choice.

Three high-order themes were confirmed as the athletes' *perceived demands* during this transition: to stay motivated; to demonstrate abilities to develop sport-specific technical skills and corresponding physical conditions; and to be able to apply the skills in their first competitions. Many athletes reported difficulty in staying motivated during the first year of specialization, because their preliminary expectations were often mistaken. For example, the young football players thought that during each practice session the coach would divide them into teams and act as a judge while they played. In other words, they expected each practice to involve continuous play. Of course this expectation was usually disconfirmed, as coaches directed the young athletes to do a lot of fitness training and technical exercises with a ball, while playing the game occupied only a portion of the training. Because this transition was studied only retrospectively, it is important to acknowledge that all the participants of the study successfully coped with it. Many athletes noticed that they felt comfortable in their sport groups because they mastered the sport easier than their teammates, received more approval and support from coaches, and were often successful in their first competitions.

Six high-order themes were identified by athletes as their *coping resources* during this transition: interest in sport in general; dreams about sport future; having fun; parental support; satisfaction with relationships in the sport group; and admiring the coach. It appears that motivational and social resources are the most important factors that keep young athletes in their chosen sports. To sum up, in this transition the young athletes prove to themselves, their parents, and coaches that they are motivated, able to learn a chosen sport, and capable of using what is learned in competitions. Athletes who fail to reach such outcomes generally drop out or change their chosen sport.

The Transition to More Intensive Training in the Chosen Sport

This transition starts when the athlete and coach decide to set sport goals and focus on achievement, which typically means implementing changes in the training schedule (typically 3-5 times per week) and content (more focus on competitive exercises in the chosen sport), and participation in higher-level competitions. In fact, this is the point when athletes enter the developmental stage of their careers, when sport begins to take up much more time and energy than before, and when they come to be considered as *prospects* in their sports.

The *perceived demands* of this transition were reflected in the following five high-order themes: to adjust to the new training regime; to improve technique/technical skills; to adjust to a higher level of competition; to become consistent in competitive performance; and to find an optimal balance between sport and studies. The essay and interview data revealed a complicated content within the first of the aforementioned demands. Many athletes experienced fear of the new training regime and loads. They often had difficulties recovering between practices and/or competitions. At the same time, they were highly motivated and even impatient to achieve their sport goals as soon as possible. They also felt the pressure of high self-expectations and the expectations of their significant others. This situation in sport, together with the obligations in the other spheres of life (such as studies), resulted in increased stress levels and often led to injuries and/or overtraining. Many athletes experienced their first serious injuries precisely during this transition, which leads to higher demands on their ability to cope. Athletes often experienced a lack of self-confidence when entering the world of higher-level competition (such as national competitions for their age groups), because the physical, technical, and tactical levels of their opponents became much higher than those of the rivals they had met previously. Athletes typically showed "ups" and "downs" in their competitive results, which stimulated them to search for ways to improve consistency in their performances.

Five high-order themes were identified in regard to the *coping resources* used during this transition: imitation of successful sport role models; interest in sport psychology; strong belief in a competence of the coach; family and school support; and satisfaction with relationships in the sport group. Again, social support appeared very important. The lack of self-confidence was compensated by the belief in the competence of the coach and the imitation of sport role models. This initial interest in sport psychology knowledge and skills, usually arising from the need to deal with anxiety, pre-competition routines, and concentration, helped young athletes feel more in control during competitions. To better manage their time between sport and studies, many athletes transferred to sport classes at their schools where schedules were adjusted to accommodate training and competitions or were admitted to sport boarding schools with their regimen dictated by sports.

Young athletes who adapted well to the new training/competition/studies regimen and were able to avoid or cope with injuries typically kept up their high aspirations to continue in their chosen sports. Those who demonstrated good performance in national- and international-level competitions for their age group eventually joined the national junior elite athletic teams, which formed a reserve for the senior national teams. In contrast, athletes who failed to cope with this transition dropped out or continued in sport on a recreational level.

The Transition from Junior to Senior Sports

The study showed that when junior athletes were successful in the national-/international-level competitions for their age group, they were often permitted to take part in senior competitions and/or to practice with a senior team. That is why the transition to senior sport and the transition to high-achievement sport, which were considered separate by the early version of the analytical model, were eventually joined into one. The transition from junior to senior sports plays the most critical role in the overall athletic career, and marks the entry into the perfection/mastery/investment stage. Athletes frequently described it as the most difficult career transition, and many of them had to acknowledge that they failed to cope with it.

The five high-order themes that defined the *demands* of this transition were: to balance sport goals with other life goals and to reorganize one's lifestyle; to search for one's individual path in sport; to cope with the pressure of selections; to win prestige among peers, judges, etc.; and to cope with possible relationship problems. According to the essay and interview data, this is the point when most junior athletes (especially those belonging to the junior elite) began to realize that, in order to succeed on the senior level, they needed to set long-term goals and make the corresponding lifestyle changes. Many put their sport goals in the forefront at the expense of other spheres of life, such as studies, professional training, work, family issues, and communication with peers. But despite all these efforts and

sacrifices, successful junior athletes often felt "lost" in senior competitions. Inevitably, their highest priorities became "getting noticed" in selections for the more prestigious competitions and earning authority among opponents, teammates, and sport professionals. Interestingly, many athletes chose to solve this problem by refusing to imitate any models and searching for an individual path/style in sport, built upon their strengths, uniqueness, or "zest." Because they take part in many competitions per season, elite junior athletes often experience a specific problem when repeatedly aiming for high performance: They often lacked the energy for the most important competitions at the end of the season. Competitiveness and rivalry increased not only in official competitions, but also within the sport groups and teams. Many athletes reported relationship problems with teammates and coaches, complaining about conflicts, misunderstandings, and intrigues. They also felt a drop in the social support and admiration they were used to as juniors.

The perceived *coping resources* outlined by athletes include: interest in scientific sport-related knowledge (sport biomechanics, physiology, psychology); summarizing and drawing upon their own sport experience; implementation of psychological strategies in competitions; learning from the mistakes of others; family and federation support. Looking through this list of themes, it is clear that the role of social resources has declined immensely when compared to the previous transitions. Instead, the athletes heavily relied on their own competencies and skills, which reflected their maturation not only as athletes but also as individuals.

The most successful athletes coped with this transition in 1-2 years or competitive seasons, but more often it took 3-4 years. Many athletes experienced this transition as a crisis: they could not cope successfully on their own and perceived a need for psychological assistance (Stambulova, 2000). However, only a small fraction of participants in the study actually collaborated with sport psychologists. In fact, this transition divided athletes into two unequal parts. The larger one stalled and moved on to recreational-level sports or terminated their participation. The smaller one continued on to the elite senior level where they were given the chance to become professional athletes.

The Transition from Amateur to Professional Sport

This transition has a clear marker: signing a professional contract. At the time of the study, professional sport was rather new to Russian athletes, and the number of participants who shared experiences related to this transition was small. Because only elite amateur athletes could become professionals, all of them were already experts in sport. But at the same time, the new Russian professionals perceived professional sport as "terra incognita."

The following five themes describe the *perceived demands* of this transition: to adjust to the terms of professional contract and a new environment; to be able to train independently; to understand the business aspects of sport; to develop a performing style attractive to spectators; and to win prestige on the professional level. When signing their first contract, all of them were afraid of being cheated. To avoid that feeling and be more in control of the subsequent contract agreements, the athletes searched for practical knowledge in justice and contract law, management, and foreign languages. Athletes who signed contracts abroad reported difficulties with cultural adaptation, communication, and social networking. At the time, Russian athletes were used to being tightly controlled and constantly directed by their coaches, so the demand to train independently and keep track of their own training schedules was new to them and required adjustment. They also learned that prestige and authority among teammates, opponents, and specialists, as well as the love of spectators, influenced their athletic success as professionals more than in amateur sports. The task of "getting noticed" came into play again, but on a much higher level. Individual style of performance, pre- and post- performance routines involving spectators, and communication with the media were used to develop a distinctive image or charisma.

Reflecting on the coping resources, all athletes noted that they relied mainly on themselves and were more selective in terms of social influences and support than previously in their careers. The following five themes describe the *perceived resources* during this transition: solid sport and life experience; awareness of one's strengths and weaknesses; compensations developed; selective use of assistance from others; and inspiration from glory. Athletes felt that they successfully coped with the transition when they were able to extend their contracts or to sign new ones.

The Transition from the Peak to the Final Stage of the Athletic Career

All athletes experience this transition, regardless of their level and status, but it is more serious for the elite and professional athletes than for those at lower levels. On the average, it occurs after 10-15 years in sport. Participants in the study reported a set of markers for the beginning of this transition, which included a plateau or a decrease in sport results; physical and psychological fatigue; anxiety about the future; health problems or consequences of former injuries; young ambitious opponents or teammates; and pressures or problems in other spheres of life (such as education, work, or family). The appearance of all or some of those symptoms stimulated athletes to think about career termination and to decide how long they wanted to stay in sport and what to do in the post-career.

The following two themes were defined as the *perceived demands* of this transition: to search for additional resources to maintain sport results on a high enough level; to plan athletic retirement. The majority of athletes did not feel ready to terminate and wanted to prolong their athletic careers. For elite athletes with their high titles and ranks, the thought of losing their leading positions in teams or ranking systems if they continued on in sport was inconceivable. So, maintaining a respectable level of achievement became a primary challenge. Veteran athletes often reported that they trained less than the younger athletes, but more efficiently.

The following three themes were identified as *perceived resources* during this transition: individualization of all aspects of sport life; solid sport and life experience; family support. Family members often satisfied the athletes' need to talk about the future and actively participated in the retirement planning. Coaches and teammates were perceived as less supportive, especially in terms of athletic retirement issues. Athletes who coped with this transition felt that their sport and life situations were under control, and they typically stayed in sport for another 2-3 years.

Athletic Career Termination and Transition to a Different Career

For every athlete, sooner or later the day comes when he or she no longer needs go to practices and prepare for competitions. The end of an athletic career is an inevitable transition, which mixes sport and non-sport contexts.

The participants of the study identified four themes as the *perceived demands* of this transition: to accept retirement and adjust to the status of a former athlete; to start/continue studies or work; to solve the identity problem; to renew the lifestyle and social network. In Russian culture, the status of former elite athletes is rather high, but it is much lower than that of active sports heroes. Therefore, former athletes needed to adjust to a substantial decrease in social recognition and support. Many threw all their energies into education or professional training to "catch up" with their non-sport peers. Starting a new professional career was not only important for making a living, but also for the development of a new personal identity. Participants of the study had a high athletic identity during their athletic careers (Hale, James, & Stambulova, 1999), and many of them kept it up in their post-career life. This may be due to the fact that a vast majority of them chose to pursue their education in sport sciences and become professional coaches or physical education teachers. Many athletes confirmed that their social life greatly changed during this transition. They often kept their sport friends, but also felt that they needed to involve more non-sport people in their social networks. Family became a very important part of their renewed lifestyle and occupied much more time than before termination in sport. For many participants, the athletic retirement transition coincided with transition into parenthood.

The following four themes were confirmed by former athletes as *perceived resources* during this transition: retirement plans; education; life interests outside of sport; family support. Athletes who received their education while still in sport planned retirement in advance, had multiple personal interests and hobbies, kept good family relationships, felt resourceful in the transition, and could adjust to their post-career in 6-12 months. About 15-20 percent experienced this transition as a crisis accompanied by unemployment, separation or divorce, health problems, alcohol abuse, and feelings of being empty, alone, and forgotten. Very few retired participants of the study searched for and received psychological assistance during this transition.

Athletic Career Transition Model

As a continuation of the study presented above, 126 crisis narratives were extracted from the athletes' essays titled, "My athletic career," to identify the symptoms of a crisis-transition and possible long-term consequences of not coping with a crisis (Stambulova, 2000, 2003). Based on these series of studies, an athletic career transition model was created (Stambulova, 2003; see also Alfermann & Stambulova, 2007) that views each transition as a process with its own demands, resources, barriers, coping, outcomes, and long-term consequences (Figure 1).

The essence of the transition process lies in coping

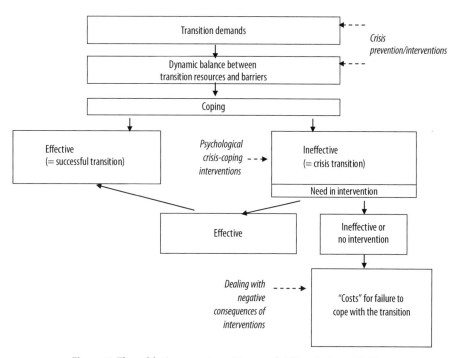

Figure 1. The athletic career transition model (Stambulova, 2003).

with a set of specific *demands* that pose a developmental conflict between "what the athlete is" and "what he or she wants or ought to be." This conflict stimulates the athlete to mobilize or develop resources to resolve it. The effectiveness of conflict resolution depends on the dynamic balance between *coping resources* and *barriers*. In this model, the "coping resources" include all internal and external factors that facilitate the coping process (knowledge, skills, personality characteristics, motivation, social and/or financial support), whereas transition "barriers" cover all internal and external factors that interfere with effective coping (lack of necessary knowledge or skills, interpersonal conflicts, absence of good conditions for training, lack of financial or social support, difficulties in combining sport with education or work). The two *outcomes* of the coping process include successful transition and crisis-transition. *Successful transition* is associated with effective coping, when the athlete is able to recruit or rapidly develop all the necessary resources to overcome transition barriers and cope with its demands. An alternative outcome is a *crisis-transition*, when the athlete is unable to cope effectively on his or her own. Research and practical experience in counseling athletes in crises (Stambulova, 2000) have identified various reasons for ineffective coping, including the athlete's low awareness of transition demands, his or her lack of resources and/or persistence of barriers, and inability to analyze the situation and make a proper decision. In order to change ineffective coping strategies, the athlete needs psychological intervention that can have an impact on the long-term *consequences of the transition*. If the intervention is effective, it is followed by a successful, but delayed, transition. If intervention is ineffective or the athlete has not received any qualified psychological assistance, the model predicts negative consequences or "costs" of the failure to cope (decline in sport performance or premature dropout, injuries, overtraining, neuroses, psychosomatic illnesses, alcohol/drug abuse, etc.). As shown in Figure 1, three kinds of interventions can be used in a career transition. *Crisis-prevention interventions* aim at preparing athletes to cope with the transition and help them develop all the necessary resources before or at the very beginning of each transition. *Crisis-coping interventions* are necessary when it is obvious that an athlete is in crisis and needs help analyzing his or her situation to find the best available way to cope. *Dealing-with-negative-consequences interventions* are typically administered when the athlete has experienced one or several of the

aforementioned "costs" of not coping with a transition. Applied issues related to optimization of athletic talent/career development and helping athletes in career transitions are presented in the next section.

Optimization of Talent/ Career Development

The Russian study presented above illustrates the athletes' perception of career transition demands and coping resources. It also reflects some features of the Russian sport system and culture, such as involvement of professional coaches from the very start of an athletic career, sport boarding schools for prospective young athletes, federation support at the peak of their career, families playing an important role throughout the careers, and availability of jobs in sport for the retired athletes (see more in Stambulova & Alfermann, in press). All of these create an environmental context for athletic talent development. It is important to note that athletes perceive different forms of social support as the most important coping resource, especially at the beginning and at the end of their athletic career. At the same time, it is interesting to consider how coaches and parents perceive athletes' transitions and what difficulties they experience with the young prospects. The author had many opportunities to talk about these issues with coaches and with athletes' parents during coaching education and sport psychology consulting in Russia (Stambulova, 1999). The three potential problems related to young prospective athletes, and suggestions on their prevention/resolution, are discussed below.

The "Rapid Progress" Problem

Coaches often shared their dilemma in dealing with young gifted athletes who demonstrate high abilities earlier than their sport peers. These athletes are "unusual" in the sense that when going through the same training program, they show more substantial progress in skills and results than their peers. These athletes are few, but they are very important for coaches. How to treat them is always a dilemma: should they be treated like the others or given more advanced and complicated tasks? In the former case, they can get bored, lose motivation, and drop out. In the latter case, there is a danger of overtraining and eventual burnout. There is no panacea for this issue, but it is possible to discern a general strategic trend: coaching as a science and an art.

"The science of coaching focuses on the use of general principles. The art of coaching is recognizing when and how to individualize these general principles" (Weinberg & Gould, 1999, p. 15). Coaches working with young talented athletes have to search carefully for optimal individual balances between performance-oriented (focused on the present) and career-oriented (focused on the future) tasks; quantity and quality of practice; competitions and recovery; values related to winning and to mastery; and preliminary plans/tactical combinations and improvisation in practice and in competition. In other words, an individual approach to the rapid progress athlete is justified, because it helps them to continue enjoying the sport and avoid burnout. It is also important to note that "natural resources" (such as quickness or coordination) only contribute to speeding up an athlete's progress during the early stages of his or her career. So, the young athletes who are used to results coming easily may experience a dissonance between their expectations and reality in the transition from junior to senior sports. Athletes' parents must be also aware of the issues relevant to the rapid progress problem. Their best possible strategy is to cooperate with the coaches and to provide optimal support and unconditional positive regard to the athletes.

The "Early Social Recognition" Problem

This problem often arises from the rapid progress problem. Young gifted athletes are "getting noticed" within their teams and in competitions. Sport specialists talk about them favorably. Coaches give positive feedback and provide support to them more often than to other athletes. In return, sport peers and teammates may feel jealous. Ambitious parents feel that they have a "gem" and dream about the young athlete's future with elevated sport titles and prize money. All in all, the athlete's significant others develop and express high expectations for the young athlete's constant progress and high results. These expectations might create a set of consequences that works as a barrier in career transitions, especially during the transition from junior to senior sports. From a performance perspective, these athletes often have over-exaggerated self-expectations, but at the same time are afraid of failure. This combination prevents them from gaining self-confidence necessary to creatively search for an individual path in senior sport. From a personal perspective, they nurture their high athletic identity at the expense of other spheres of life, which might create seri-

ous problems in case of injury and premature dropout. From a social perspective, the recognized young athletes feel like "stars" in their groups or teams, but they are also afraid to lose this status. As a result, they may spend too much energy on maintaining it. Parents who invested their time, energy, and money expect a return. As one figure skater's mother pointed out in a communication with the author:

> I brought my daughter to this big city from a province. I left everything behind—my husband, my job, my relatives and friends—to provide my child with the best possible conditions to develop her athletic talent. I can say that I gave her my all. Now it is her turn to give back to me. She must do everything to become an elite and professional skater.

Unfortunately, this girl failed her mother's expectations because of an eating disorder followed by a premature dropout.

It is difficult to prevent the early social recognition itself when young athletes show impressive results. But it is possible to reduce or to minimize its negative consequences. Coaches have to search for an optimal balance between cooperation and competition in youth teams/groups, emphasizing cooperation and using less comparison and more personal-referenced criteria in their evaluation of athletes. It is also important to ensure that a "star" gets more popularity but no more privileges than any other team member when following basic group norms (Stambulova, 1999). Parents should again provide the unconditional positive regard and optimal support to the athletes, protecting them from becoming "public personas" before they are ready.

The "One-Sided Development" Problem

This problem can be seen as a logical consequence of not coping with the rapid progress and early social recognition problems. Young prospect athletes with high and exclusive athletic identities often experience a disharmony in their development: They mature as athletes much earlier than as individuals. This is particularly obvious during the transition from junior to senior sports. There are many examples of 14- to 16-year-old gymnasts, swimmers, divers, and figure skaters, who not only participate in the highest level of senior competitions—but also win them. Winning rapidly propels them to the top in amateur sport, and many of them rush to sign professional contracts. Moorman (2000) described this situation in the example of Oksana Baiul—the Ukrainian figure skater who won the Olympics at the age of 16 and immediately moved on to professional sport in the USA. As Moorman pointed out:

> She experienced many problems, not only regarding her skating … but in her personal life as well. When she won the Olympics she had the figure of a young girl, e.g., skinny. When she became professional her body changed. She gained some weight when she matured and she did not look that skinny anymore. Those "normal" body changes now caused her problems with triple jumps. Several injuries followed. The psychological transition from childhood to adulthood could be called rushed. Being a professional now, she had to behave as if she were an adult and in many cases she was treated as such. She obviously could not cope with this transition. She had a car accident, for instance, and it turned out that she had been drunk while driving. The reasons for this tragedy were evident. She simply was not ready yet for this transition, psychologically or physically. (p. 605)

Several applied issues are relevant in this case and in general for prevention of one-sided development and related problems. First of all, cooperative efforts of sport managers, coaches, parents, and sport psychology consultants are needed to nurture athletic talents properly. Second, all significant others involved should strive for a holistic view of an athlete and realize that sport is only one part of the athlete's larger life. Athletes' interests, competencies, and activities outside of sport enrich their personalities and should be supported. Third, it is beneficial to prepare athletes in advance for normative career transitions by making them aware of the forthcoming transition demands, and helping them recruit/develop the necessary resources in advance. It is also important to foresee the potential transition barriers and find ways to eliminate them. Fourth, professional psychological assistance should be sought not only to foster the athletes' readiness to a career transition (Alfermann, Stambulova, & Zemaityte, 2004), but also to help the athletes overcome crisis-transitions once they pass beyond prevention (Stambulova, 2000).

Career Assistance

Psychological career services around the world (lifestyle management programs, life/career skills programs, and career assistance programs; see Wylleman, Theeboom, & Lavallee, 2004 for an overview) combine workshops, seminars, educational modules, individual counseling, and mental training in helping athletes to successfully self-actualize in sport and adjust to the post-career. The philosophy behind these services can be summarized as follows: A *whole career approach* helps athletes cope with both normative and non-normative transitions throughout the whole course of an athletic career. A *whole person approach* helps athletes deal not only with athletic but also non-athletic transitions in psychological, psychosocial, and academic-vocational development (Wylleman & Lavallee, 2004). A *developmental approach* provides links between past career experiences, the present situation, and the athlete's perceived future. It helps athletes to be proactive and make decisions for the future by selecting ways to cope with the current situation that may also help them prepare for the future demands. An *activity-specific approach* takes into account not just the common but also the sport-specific demands in each athletic transition. For example, during the transition from junior to senior level, representatives of team sports can expect an increase in social demands, while representatives of complex coordination sports (gymnastics, figure skating) should focus on increasing the complexity of their performance routines. A *culture-specific approach* helps athletes adjust within a particular sport system and culture. An *individual approach* focuses on the athlete's perception of the transition and his or her idiosyncratic internal/external resources and barriers. A *transferable skills approach* encourages athletes to develop mental skills applicable both within and outside sport (e.g., stress/time/energy management). Finally, an *empowerment approach* teaches athletes to develop their own coping resources/strategies to become more autonomous after psychological interventions and less dependent on consultants and their services.

Conclusions and Future Directions

This chapter is focused on a relatively new perspective on talent development in sport. This perspective relates to career development, with an emphasis on career transitions as turning points/phases in this process. Athletic career development is viewed as a broader context for talent development, whereas an athlete's talent is considered not only as a set of motor skills and qualities, but also as the ability to develop and effectively use resources to overcome transition demands inside and outside of sport.

Despite the traditionally high interest in this topic by sport scientists and practitioners, there are still many questions left unanswered and many aspects left unclear. First, more work is needed on the terminology to prevent the confusion of the multi-meaning term *talent*. Second, more studies should be done on the within athletic career transitions and parallel transitions in other spheres of life. Another promising research direction is the talent development environment, including coaches, peers, families, school, sport system, mass media, and national culture. Additionally cross-cultural studies may also be of interest. Finally, more attention should be paid to career issues in applied sport psychology education, and more career assistance services should be offered around the world to help athletes realize their full potential in sport and in life.

References

Alfermann, D., & Stambulova, N. (2007). Career transitions and career termination. In G. Tenenbaum & R. C. Eklund (Eds.), *Handbook of sport psychology* (3rd ed., pp. 712-736). New York: Wiley.

Alfermann, D., Stambulova, N., & Zemaityte, A. (2004). Reactions to sports career termination: A cross-national comparison of German, Lithuanian, and Russian athletes. *Psychology of Sport & Exercise, 5/1,* 61-75.

Bloom, B. S. (Ed.). (1985). *Developing talent in young people.* New York: Ballantine Books.

Côté, J. (1999). The influence of the family in the development of talent in sport. *The Sport Psychologist, 13,* 395-417.

Côté, J., Baker, J., & Abernethy, B. (2007). Practice and play in the development of sport expertise. In G. Tenenbaum & R. C. Eklund (Eds.), *Handbook of sport psychology* (3rd ed., pp. 184-202). New York: Wiley.

Durand-Bush, N., & Salmela, J. H. (2001). Development of talent in sport. In R. N. Singer, H. A. Hausenblas, & C. M. Janelle (Eds.), *Handbook of sport psychology* (2nd ed., pp. 269-289). New York: Wiley.

Hale, B. D., James, B., & Stambulova, N. (1999). Determining the dimensionality of athletic identity: A "Herculean" cross-cultural undertaking. *International Journal of Sport Psychology, 30,* 83-100.

Hanin, Y., & Stambulova, N. (2004). Sport psychology, overview. In C. Spielberger (Ed.), *Encyclopedia of applied psychology* (Vol. 3, pp. 463-477). New York: Elsevier.

Henriksen, K., Roessler, K. K., & Stambulova, N. (2007). Talent development environment in sport: An explorative case study based on the system's theory framework. Proceedings of the 12th European Congress of Sport Psychology, Halkidiki, Greece.

Feldhusen, J. F. (2004). Gifted students. In C. Spielberger (Ed.), *Encyclopedia of applied psychology* (Vol. 2, pp. 105-108). New York: Elsevier.

Maes, M. (2004). Talent and ethics. In Y. Vanden Auweele (Ed.), *Ethics in youth sport—Analyses and recommendations* (pp. 117-126). Ghent, Belguim: Lannoo Campus.

Martindale, R. J., Collins, D., & Abraham, A. (2007). Effective talent development: The elite coach perspective in UK sport. *Journal of Applied Sport Psychology, 19,* 187-206.

Moorman, P. P. (2000). The diathesis-stress paradigm for better understanding of the complexities of athletes' crises. *International Journal of Sport Psychology, 31,* 602-609.

Salmela, J. H. (1994). Phases and transitions across sports careers. In D. Hackfort (Ed.), *Psycho-social issues and interventions in elite sport* (pp. 11-28). Frankfurt: Lang.

Stambulova, N. (1994). Developmental sports career investigations in Russia: A post- perestroika analysis. *The Sport Psychologist, 8,* 221-237.

Stambulova, N. (1995). Sports career transitions of Russian athletes. In R. Vanfraechem-Raway & Y. Vanden Auweele (Eds.), *Proceedings of the IXth European Congress of Sport Psychology* (pp. 867-872). Brussels, Belgium: ATM.

Stambulova, N. (1999). *Psihologiya sportivnoi kariery* [Psychology of the athletic career]. St.-Petersburg: Career Promotion Centre.

Stambulova, N. (2000). Athletes' crises: A developmental perspective. *International Journal of Sport Psychology, 31,* 584-601.

Stambulova, N. (2003). Symptoms of a crisis-transition: A grounded theory study. In N. Hassmén (Ed.), *SIPF Yearbook 2003* (pp. 97-109). Örebro: Örebro University.

Stambulova, N., & Alfermann, D. (in press). Putting culture into context: Cultural and cross-cultural perspectives in career development and transition research and practice. *International Journal of Sport and Exercise Psychology.*

Wylleman, P., & Lavallee, D. (2004). A developmental perspective on transitions faced by athletes. In M. Weiss (Ed.), *Developmental sport and exercise psychology: A lifespan perspective* (pp. 507-527). Morgantown, WV: Fitness Information Technology.

Wylleman, P., Theeboom, M., & Lavallee, D. (2004). Successful athletic careers. In C. Spielberger (Ed.), *Encyclopedia of applied psychology* (Vol. 3, pp. 511-517). New York: Elsevier.

CHAPTER 8

Interdisciplinary Teaching, Goal Orientation, Self-Determination, and Responsibility in Life

ATHANASIOS G. PAPAIOANNOU AND DIMITRIOS MILOSIS

Sport psychology aims at helping individuals to excel in sport and life (Cox, 1994). Indeed, many of the world's greatest coaches are committed to teaching their athletes how to excel not only in sport but in life as well (Gould, Collins, Lauer, & Chung, 2006). However, while the subject of performance enhancement strategies is a hot topic in sport psychology research, strategies aiming at enhancing personal development and life skills have been studied less often (Gould et al., 2006). Nelsen, Lott, and Glenn (1997) argued that self-discipline, social interest, and sense of responsibility are essential skills that enable people to act effectively in life. Hellison (1995) suggested a curriculum that primarily focuses on the development of youngsters' responsibility through physical activity involvement. Others suggested that holistic physical activity programs should be employed for the development of the emotional, spiritual, and intellectual self as well as the physical self (Noddings, 1992). The present chapter describes an interdisciplinary program in physical education aim-

ing at the development of personal development goals in life, self-determination in life, general self-esteem, self-perception of honesty, and positive attitudes toward responsible behaviors in sport events. The present authors have previously reported on the effects of this intervention on achievement goals, intrinsic motivation, self-perceptions, and satisfaction in physical activity and school contexts, and more specifically in physical education, math, and language classes (Milosis & Papaioannou, 2007).

At the core of this intervention is the creation of a positive motivational climate aiming at the development of adaptive goal orientations for participants. Motivational climate is defined as a situational-induced environment directing the goals of an action in achievement situations (Ames, 1992a). A mastery climate emphasizes effort, competence development, and optimum challenge for all individuals (Nicholls, 1989). A performance approach climate emphasizes outperforming others and high normative ability. Finally, a performance avoidance climate directs individuals' efforts toward avoidance of exhibition of low ability (Papaioannou, Tsigilis, Kosmidou, & Milosis, 1997). These climate dimensions influence the development of individuals' predisposition toward pursuing mastery, performance approach, and performance avoidance goals, respectively (Papaioannou, Ampatzoglou, Kalogiannis, & Sagovits, in press). A large number of studies imply that mastery goals are adaptive and a performance avoidance climate is maladaptive for achievement in school and sport (e.g., Conroy, Elliot, & Hofer, 2003; Duda, 2005; Elliot, 2005), while many authors believe that performance approach goals also should be discouraged, particularly because they lead to antisocial behavior (e.g., Duda, Olson, & Templin, 1991; Kavussanu & Ntoumanis, 2003).

Relevant to the present study is the effect of goal orientation on intrinsic-extrinsic motivation and self-determination. Deci and Ryan (1985) suggested that reasons for action vary in degree of self-determination. In the high-low self-determination continuum intrinsic reasons for action lies as the upper-highest level, followed by identified, introjected, and external, respectively, while amotivation lies at the bottom-lowest level of self-determined regulation. Intrinsic reasons emerge in activities that are undertaken for intrinsic pleasure and satisfaction. Identified regulation takes place when an action is a means to an end—it is not enjoyable but is considered important or the individual feels no pressure to accomplish it. Introjected regulation takes place when the individual feels internal pressure to do the activity. External reasons for action are pressures from the environment such as external demands from teachers, supervisors, etc. Amotivation emerges when there is lack of intention and control for an observed action; individuals do not know why they are doing the activity and feel helpless while they are doing it. Theory and research imply that personal improvement goals are positively linked with high self-determination, intrinsic motivation, and identified regulation, but ego goals are positively linked with low self-determination, external regulation, and amotivation (Ntoumanis, 2001; Standage, Duda, & Ntoumanis, 2003).

Although goal orientations are affected by a particular context, such as sport, individuals bring into a situation their own goal orientations, which have been formatted in other settings, such as school or family (Papaioannou et al., in press). Taking into consideration that goal orientations generalize across different domains (Duda & Nicholls, 1992), Papaioannou (1999) suggested that individuals hold global goal orientations in life that predispose them to adopt the same pattern of goals when they enter into a new situation. Imagine two children with similar physical abilities who start a sport on the same day. One has a history of pursuing mastery in math and language classes, in jigsaw puzzles, in drawing, and in theatrical performances, but the other has a history of not pursuing mastery in any setting. Our prediction is that at least in the first few weeks the first child will be more eager to pursue sport competence improvement than the second. The coach should be more patient with the second child and always provide opportunities for improvement in order to help this child develop mastery orientation in the sport.

The first child probably has a stronger orientation toward personal development in life than the second. The question then is whether we can change global goal orientations through training. Global psychological constructs such as global self-esteem (Marsh & Yeung, 1998) and global self-determination (Guay, Mageau, & Vallerand, 2003) are determined by the same constructs (i.e., self-perceptions and self-determination) that operate in a variety of specific contexts. Accordingly, multidisciplinary interventions should be more effective in changing individuals' global goal orientations than interventions focusing on a particular domain. Recently, using interdisciplinary teaching in a physical education setting, we were successful in altering goal orientations and self-esteem in the contexts of physical education, math, and language classes (Milosis & Papaioannou, 2007). In the present study we focus on the effects of this program on global goal orientations, global self-determination, and global self-esteem. We present more extensively our intervention on responsibility goals and outcomes and we present findings concerning the effects of this program on attitudes toward violence in sport events. Below we describe the theoretical model that was used in the present intervention. Then the intervention is briefly portrayed followed by the results and a discussion.

Multidimensional Model of Goal Orientations (MMGO)

Based on theories suggesting that goals vary in levels of abstraction (Carver & Sheier, 1998; Vallacher & Wegner, 1987), and following Vallerand's (1997) suggestions that motivational constructs such as intrinsic-extrinsic motivation have an hierarchical structure, Papaioannou (1999) proposed a taxonomy of goal orientations at four levels of generality (Figure 1):

(1) Goal orientations generally in life are at the highest order level of generality;

(2) At the next lower level are goal orientations that generalize across life settings but are specific to a particular domain of human action (e.g., achievement, responsibility);

(3) Even lower are contextual goal orientations that are shaped by the features of the particular life setting (e.g., sport, school, and work); and

(4) At the lowest level are situational goal orientations (i.e., at the here and now), which are largely affected by the particular situation at a particular moment.

At the highest level of generality, the following definition of goals has been adopted. *Personal development goal* directs individuals at improving their qualities across a variety of actions and life contexts. *Ego-strengthening goal* directs individuals to gain a positive evaluation of their qualities from others. An *ego-protection goal* connotes attempts to avoid negative judgments of one's qualities from others. Finally, particularly in collectivistic cultures, individuals pursue *social approval goals* through the adoption of various actions across different life settings.

This taxonomy is based on the assumption that goal orientations have implications for achieving and non-achieving behaviors, such as responsibility, morality, health-related behaviors, etc. Based on this assumption, we set goals in the present study for improvement in both the achievement and responsibility domains.

The next premise of this model concerns the antecedents and consequences of goal orientations. The motivational climate created by coaches, parents, peers, teachers, idols, media, and the general culture has an influence on individuals' goal adoption at different levels of generality. Everyday interaction with social agents typically affects goal orientations at the situational and contextual levels. Social agents, such as parents, who educate youth how to behave across different contexts, implicitly or explicitly influence children's global goal orientations. Culture also affects global goal orientations, as was shown in a recent cross-cultural study (Papaioannou, 2006).

The adoption of a particular goal orientation leads to specific cognitions, emotions, and behaviors. For

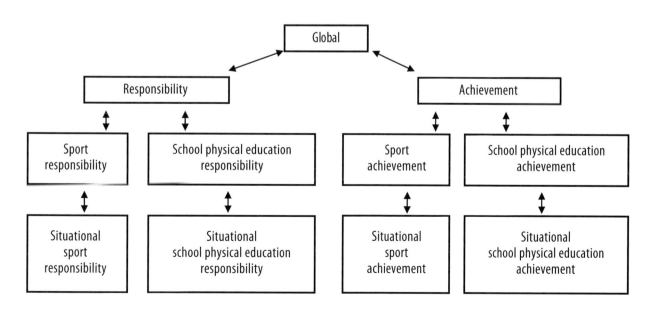

Figure 1. Hierarchical levels of generality.

example, in physical activity contexts, personal development goals facilitate positive emotions and efficient cognitive strategies such as self-monitoring and planning. On the other hand, ego goal orientations are not connected with positive emotions but with superficial thinking and impression management (Ntoumanis & Biddle, 1999; Ommudsen, 2003; Theodosiou & Papaioannou, 2006). We also know that only personal development goals facilitate sport and exercise involvement, which in turn reinforces even further the adoption of personal improvement in sport (Papaioannou, Bebetsos, Theodorakis, Christodoulidis, & Kouli, 2006).

The MMGO and Interdisciplinary Teaching

Skills such as cooperation, communication, planning, self-monitoring, evaluation, and corrective intervention strategies determine one's progress across different disciplines, and therefore they are called interdisciplinary skills (Greek Ministry of Education, 2003). Others call them life skills because they facilitate personal growth and success in life (Danish & Donohue, 1995). Because sport is an achievement domain, these authors suggested that sport can teach children how to transfer these aptitudes to other life contexts: the ability to perform under pressure, to meet deadlines and challenges, to set goals, and to handle both success and failure (Danish & Nellen, 1997). Still, others believe that sport can teach skills that are connected with character values such as responsibility, self-control, courage, and persistence (Klieber & Roberts, 1981), which are also considered prerequisites for success in life (Nelsen et al., 1997).

The MMGO is a useful theoretical framework for teaching all the aforementioned skills, because social environments emphasizing personal improvement goals are perceived to have positive association with cooperation, communication, planning, self-monitoring, subjective evaluation of success and failure, self-discipline, responsibility and persistence (see Duda, 1989a, b; Ommundsen, 2003; Papaioannou, 1998; Solmon & Lee, 1997; Theodosiou & Papaioannou, 2006). Moreover, social environments emphasizing personal improvement goals but not ego-strengthening goals are expected to increase athletes' self-determination (Ntoumanis, 2001) and moral functioning (Kavussanu & Roberts, 2001).

The MMGO takes into account all social environments affecting the formation of individuals' goal orientations in a particular context as well as across contexts (Papaioannou 2006; Papaioannou et al., in press). A practical implication of the MMGO for social agents (e.g., coaches) is to encourage adaptive goal orientations, not only in these contexts but in other life settings as well. This implies that coaches, teachers, and parents should also encourage personal improvement goal adoption and discourage ego-protection goal adoption at a high level of generality. Indeed, the motto of the present intervention was "By improving myself everywhere I will live better." This motto reinforces the necessity to pursue personal improvement and provides a reason for high effort across a variety of learning tasks, school subjects, and life settings. In other words, the motto emphasizes both the goal and its outcome at the global level of generality.

Of course, most of our intervention focused on personal improvement in specific settings. Based on the recommendations of social learning theory emphasizing enactive learning (Bandura, 1986), we first provided a wealth of task-involving experiences in physical education, and then we asked students to transfer what they learned to other life contexts. In all physical education classes we promoted task-involving activities, personal goal setting, and cognitive strategies that facilitate task-involvement. In the final minutes of each class we discussed how these goals and strategies could be used in math and Greek language, as well as and in terms of student responsibility in home, school, and sport settings. Then, we asked the students to set goals and employ strategies for personal improvement in these contexts. A few days or weeks after the practice of personal improvement goals and strategies in other life settings, we reviewed with the students their experiences, the pros and cons of applying personal improvement goals and strategies in these life settings, the barriers that emerged, and the coping skills that were employed to overcome obstacles and mistakes, and then we asked the students to revise their goals and strategies and apply them again. This process allowed us to reinforce the importance of the motto "by improving myself everywhere I will live better."

In addition to global goal orientations we tried to affect global self-determination. As described below, we created conditions where students were asked to make decisions concerning learning and behaving in school, in sport, at home, and in life. We also anticipated that our emphasis on personal development goals would have positive effects on global intrinsic motivation and global self-determination, and negative effects on external regulation and amotivation at the global level of generality (Vallerand, 1997).

Global self-esteem was another focus of our study. We expected that an increase in personal development goals in life would have positive effects on global self-esteem, because students adopting personal criteria of success across different domains have a sense of accomplishment and personal worth when they register personal progress (Covingthon, 1992). Take the example of the physical education setting. If a strong emphasis is given to personal improvement, all students will feel successful as long as they improve their skills and personal performances. This will increase their self-worth and perception of physical ability. If students perceive a similar environment across settings, then they will have multiple experiences of success and personal progress, and all dimensions of self-concept (e.g., physical, verbal, and social) will improve; this will eventually increase their global self-esteem. Indeed, we reported elsewhere that the present intervention had positive effects on physical and verbal self-concept as well as math ability (Milosis & Papaioannou, 2007).

In the same chapter we also reported the effects of this program on self-determination in sport contexts and on goal orientations and satisfaction in achievement domains such as physical education, math, and language classes (Milosis & Papaioannou, 2007). Here we will report findings concerning non-achievement behaviors, such as violence in sport-related events. We predicted that our emphasis on responsibility goals would have a negative effect on attitudes toward sport-related violence.

Responsibility and the MMGO

The purpose of education is to prepare children for responsible citizenship, because societies consisting of socially responsible citizens function in a positive manner. Respect and responsibility are the two fundamental moral values that schools should teach. These values are necessary for healthy personal development, caring interpersonal relationships, a human and democratic society, and a just and peaceful world. Respect means showing regard for the worth of someone or something. It takes three major forms: respect for oneself, respect for other people, and respect for all forms of life and the environment that sustains them. Responsibility literally means "ability to respond." It means orienting toward others, paying attention to them, and actively responding to their needs. Responsibility emphasizes our positive obligations to care for each other (Lickona, 1991, 1997) and to act on the regard for the worth of someone or something (Morris, 2003). Lickona pointed out some specific values such as honesty, fairness, tolerance, prudence, self-discipline, helpfulness, compassion, cooperation, courage, and a host of democratic values as forms of respect and/or responsibility or aids to acting respectfully and responsibly (Lickona, 1991).

Hellison (1996) described two forms of responsibility: personal and social. Personal responsibility refers to individuals who are willing to try and experience new things, work on their own, and develop and carry out a plan for themselves that will enhance their well being. Social responsibility refers to individuals who respect the rights and feelings of others and are sensitive and responsive to the well being of others. Hellison (1995, 1996) developed a model to help students and young athletes improve responsibility in physical activity domains. His model consists of a progression of levels of responsibility:

0 = Irresponsibility, defined as neglect for the rights of others; students denying personal responsibility and blaming others for their behavior.

1 = Respect, defined as controlling one's behavior to avoid interference with the rights of others.

2 = Participation, defined as respect for others and willing involvement in physical activity under the direction of the teacher or coach.

3 = Self-direction, defined as working effectively without supervision, which involves planning and execution of one's own physical activity program.

4 = Caring, defined as sensitivity and responsiveness to the well being of others, including cooperating, giving support, showing concern, and helping others.

5 = Outside the gym, defined as trying the levels 2-4 out of the gym, in the classroom, on the playground and street, and at home.

Hellison's program helps children to classify their behaviors according to these levels through teaching (e.g., role playing) and self-reflection in real life physical activity settings, and then to set goals for improvement from lower levels (0-1) to higher levels (2-5) of responsibility. We have shown that these levels of responsibility are parallel to the levels of self-determination described by Deci and Ryan (1985), and that they are strongly connected with goal orientations and motivational climate in physical education (Papaioannou, 1998). Specifically, the lower levels of self-determination are connected with ego goals and ego-oriented climates, but the higher levels of responsibility are positively linked with personal improvement goals and mastery-oriented climates. Hellison's model also fits nicely with the MMGO because it clarifies how to set personal development goals in the responsibility domain in sport settings and how to transfer these goals to other life settings; in turn, this model serves to reinforce the importance of pursuing personal improvement goals in both achievement and responsibility domains, and in life in general. Accordingly, Hellison's model was presently employed to promote responsibility in physical education, in other school subjects, in the home, and in sport-related events.

Due to the large number of dependent variables (see also Milosis & Papaioannou, 2007), the increased number of resources required for the intervention, and the complexity of the intervention itself, we did not use any direct measure of responsibility. However, we examined the effects of the intervention on the honesty component of self-concept (Marsh, Parker, & Barnes, 1985) and students' attitudes toward sport-related violence. The latter was assessed based on Ajzen's theory of planned behavior (1988), which suggests that the best social-cognitive predictor of a specific behavior is intention, followed by perception of control of this behavior and attitudes toward this behavior. In previous studies involving large representative samples of Greek adolescents, we found that intentions, perceived behavioral control, and attitudes toward sport-related violence are positively connected with sport involvement and particularly with health-risks such as smoking and drug use (e.g., Papaioannou, Karastogiannidou, & Theodorakis, 2004). Hence, coaches and physical education teachers should teach children how to stay away from antisocial behaviors in sport events.

Method

Participants

Participants in the study were 292 (n = 162 male, n = 130 female) first-year students in the first year in junior high school (aged 12.38 ± .68) from six schools located in different areas of a Greek urban area. Ninety-nine students from four classes comprised the experimental group. These were taught by a specially-trained physical education (PE) teacher for a six-month period (each student had three school classes per week). The teacher had completed his master's on motivation in PE and the present study was part of his doctoral dissertation. The control group was comprised of 193 students from eight classes who were taught the typical PE subject by three male and four female teachers.

Measures

A researcher (someone other than the PE teacher) who applied the intervention program visited the schools the first week of the academic year and one week after the completion of the intervention and collected the self-reports. All students were told that the aim of the study was to examine the validity of questionnaires assessing motivation, attitudes, and self-concept in different domains of human action. All students completed questionnaires assessing: (a) four global goal orientations (Personal Improvement, Ego-Strengthening, Ego-Protection, and Social Approval, in life in general) (Papaioannou, 2006; Papaioannou, Milosis, Kosmidou, & Tsigilis, 2002); (b) global Intrinsic-Extrinsic Motivation and Amotivation (Global Motivational Scale) (Guay, Blais, Vallerand, & Pelletier, 1996; Guay et al., 2003); (c) general Self and Honesty-Trustworthiness scales of the Multidimensional Self-Concept (Marsh et al., 1985); and (d) Attitudes, Intentions and Perceived Behavioral Control toward involvement in violent actions in sport-related events (Papaioannou et al., 2004; Theodorakis, Papaioannou, & Karastogiannidou, 2004). Students responded to items on a five-point scale (I absolutely agree = 5, I absolutely disagree = 1) for global goal orientations and motivation, and on a six-point scale (false = 1, true = 6) for self-concept. For the assessment of attitudes students indicated their responses to the statement, "For me to participate in a violent act in a sport-related event during the next 12 months is…" on a 7-point scale consisting of four sets of opposite adjectives (good = 7, bad = 1; healthy = 7, unhealthy = 1; useful = 7, useless =1;

pleasant =7, unpleasant =1). Two items were used to assess intentions: "I intend/I am determined to be involved in violent acts in sport-related events." Responses were rated on a 7-point scale (likely = 7, unlikely = 1; absolutely yes = 7, absolutely no = 1). Finally, students responded to three items assessing perceived control: "For me to participate in a violent act in a sport-related event during the next 12 months is…" and responses were indicated on 7-point scales (difficult = 7, easy = 1; highly probable = 7, hardly probable = 1). After the initial completion of the questionnaires, the students of the experimental group were informed about the program that was going to be taught that year, the purpose and the aim of it, its main characteristics, and its importance. For the assessment of the self-determination score, we used the formula commonly used in self-determination theory literature [(2 * intrinsic) + identified – external – (2 * amotivation)] (e.g., Guay et al., 2003).

Procedure

The present study targeted both goals and their outcomes at different levels of generality (see Figure 2). The intervention predominantly tried to promote personal improvement goals and its outcomes in three domains of human action, that is, the (a) social domain, (b) health domain, and (c) achievement domain (in the contexts of PE, math, and Greek language). This emphasis on personal development created a climate that reduced social evaluation concerns and, as a consequence, did not provide incentives to students to pursue ego-oriented goals. Interdisciplinary teaching was employed to influence goal adoption, self-concept, and outcomes across different school subjects and life contexts and to strengthen their horizontal links.

Improvement in the Social Domain

To facilitate improvement in the social domain, we adopted the model of Hellison (1995). Contents from other models or methods were also utilized (Kirschenbaum, 1995; Lickona, 1991; Nelsen et al., 1997).

Intervention on social goals: Responsibility domain. This intervention benefited from Kirschenbaum's (1995) suggestion that educational approaches and techniques that help young people learn to be better goal-setters contribute to values in education. Successful goal-setters are going to be more effective in their personal lives and will contribute more to their work setting and community. A part of the goal setting program described below focused on the improvement of students' responsibility. In addition, students were taught the levels of responsibility suggested by Hellison (1995), that is, (0) irresponsibility, (I) respecting the rights and feelings of others,

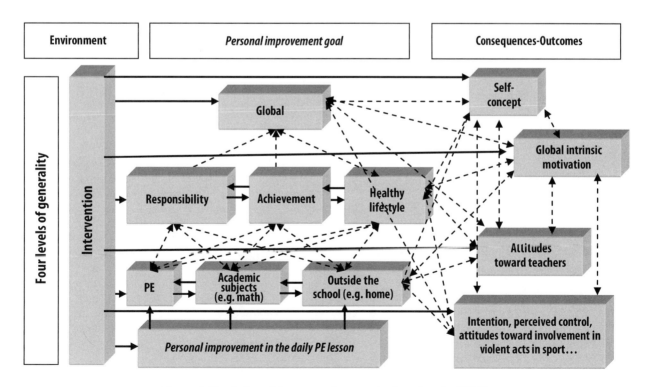

Figure 2. The design of the present intervention based on the MMGO.

(II) participation and effort, (III) self-direction, (IV) caring about and helping others, (V) outside the gym. They then were encouraged to move from lower-order levels to higher-order levels of responsibility.

Intervention on outcomes in the social domain:

(1) Promotion of responsible behavior. A constructive discipline atmosphere of caring based on kindness and firmness, dignity, and mutual respect was created through the following content (Kirschenbaum, 1995; Lickona, 1991; Nelsen et al., 1997):

- At the beginning of the school year, after a discussion between the PE teacher and the students, a list of the rights and responsibilities of every student in the PE class was developed. The list was hung up on the bulletin board, and all students agreed not to infringe upon the rights of their classmates.

- Students were involved in activities requiring them to set rules and take responsibility for keeping them. Through this process the students understood that rules and laws exist not just for their own sake, but to help achieve mutual respect, fair play, and other values that are deemed important by society.

- In the beginning of the year reasonable and fair consequences for rule-breaking were introduced. In some cases the consequences were set in cooperation with the students.

- In some instances troublemakers were advised to choose between different responses (for example, a student was told "It's not okay to hurt your classmate. You can apologize now or take some time to cool off and put this on the agenda for the next class meeting.").

- Appropriate behavior was reinforced.

- Self-monitoring was reinforced aiming to exercise self-discipline. Students were encouraged to observe, assess, and record on a personal form the occasions of their responsible behaviors predetermined by the teacher, and then to set a goal for improvement in the responsibility domain for the next month, through the self-regulation program described below.

- Students were involved in the solution of discipline problems individually or in groups by being given the chance to listen, express their opinion, and make comments. Through this process we expected them to cultivate thinking and communicating skills, because these are considered important parts of values education (Kirschenbaum, 1995). Class meetings were organized in order to handle critical issues and concerns such as problems that need to be solved, interpersonal conflicts to work out, or discussions that need to be made.

- A supportive atmosphere was created through an emphasis on cooperation and inclusion and by discouraging negative comments, non-constructive criticism, and social comparison.

- The teacher used reminders to always sustain positive attitudes and expectations toward all students and to act as a model of support, fair treatment, respect for others, etc.

(2) Moral thinking. Interdisciplinary educational activities focusing on the development of the ideals of fair play (respect for the rules, respect for officials and their decisions, respect for the opponent, providing all individuals with an equal chance to participate, and maintaining self-control at all times) were used (Commission for Fair Play, 1990). Teaching strategies focused primarily on dialogue and problem-solving tasks associated with the identification and resolution of moral conflicts and moral dilemmas. Students were encouraged to use the problem solving strategy (problem, alternatives, consequences, and solution) to resolve conflict situations. They were also provided with opportunities to discuss questions about conflicts they resolved, strategies they used, and occasions that they lost their self-control (Gibbons & Ebbeck, 1997). In playing conditions, students were involved in situations where they faced moral dilemmas and were asked to solve moral disputes by playing different roles each time; for example, a player who made a violation of the rules that the referee didn't realize or a player or team that was judged unfairly.

Hypothetical moral dilemmas were discussed in the classroom, particularly when the PE lesson couldn't be held on the playground due to bad weather conditions. According to Kirschenbaum (1995), sometimes in actual situations, especially when peer pressure may be operating, people forget to examine the moral dimensions of a problem and make a choice purely based on immediate self-interest. By presenting students with hypothetical choices, we attempted to give them an opportunity to think about difficult situations and explore possible solutions when it doesn't really "count." With input from the PE teacher and their classmates, we tried to assist students to reaffirm values and moral principles and to get in the habit of applying moral criteria in real-life dilemmas. The students, in teams of four to six, were given a hypothetical moral dilemma to discuss for a few minutes and were expected to try to reach an agreement about what they would do in that situation. Following this, the entire class engaged in a discussion expounding their opinions according to the choices that were made. For example: "Your best friends invite you to watch a soccer match of your favorite team. You know that your friends enjoy going to a place where fanatic supporters sometimes congregate and usually participate in violent actions during the match. What is your choice, to go along with them, despite running the risk of getting into trouble, or to miss the match if you cannot persuade them to go to a more peaceful place?" or, "Your best friends smoke cigarette and you don't. They pressure you to start smoking in order to be an acceptable member of the group. What is your choice, to start smoking or to lose your friends in case you cannot persuade them to quit smoking?"

(3) *Assignments.* Some home assignments were given aiming at the cultivation of responsible behavior. For example, students had to collect articles from sport newspapers describing events of sport violence, or articles that implicitly or explicitly encouraged aggression against the referee or against the fans of an opposite team. Then for the same situations they had to provide alternative solutions or to restructure the writing of the articles, in order to prohibit sport violence or aggression.

(4) *Responsible behavior in after-school physical activities.* It has been supported that extracurricular participation in teams, clubs, and sport activities provides countless opportunities for values' education (Kirschenbaum, 1995). In the present program,

students were encouraged to come voluntarily to school in the afternoons and to participate in a variety of physical activities. The PE teacher was at school three afternoons per week to supervise the work done by the students. As the students arrived at the school, they were reminded that the aim of their participation in these activities was to improve in the health and responsibility domain. For this purpose, the students were encouraged to exercise and to choose activities, space, equipment, and teams. Also, they were reminded to perform the skills being taught in the class (e.g., development and program application of physical condition, cooperation, problem-solving, conflict resolution, goal-setting, self-control, self-monitoring, and self-talk). When necessary, the teacher intervened to help students attain their goals. At the end of the practice session a brief discussion followed with the students referring to the degree of their goal accomplishments, and the difficulties they encountered and the strategies they used to resolve them. Students were also encouraged to participate in physical activities during breaks between academic subjects, and they were provided with the necessary equipment (e.g., balls, racquets, ropes). During these activities the teacher reinforced responsibility by asking the students to follow rules set in common (e.g., play safely, return sport material back in place, and involve others in the games). Finally, special emphasis was put on the generalization of these skills outside the school.

(5) *Parental involvement.* Students were encouraged to persuade and motivate their parents to participate together with them in physical activities on the weekends. The students were deemed responsible for planning and implementing an appropriate program according to the needs of their parents. We did this because values education and moral education are considered a joint responsibility of the family, the school, and the institutions of the community (Kirschenbaum, 1995).

The PE teacher helped students to attract the interest of their parents. Communication with parents started at the beginning of the school year. Initially, a letter was sent to parents outlining the program, its aim, and the PE teacher's expectations, asking them to commit to contributing to the success of the program through their active support and involvement. Letters were also sent whenever necessary to keep parents informed. Parents were invited to the school one afternoon to attend a lecture on motivation, goal orientation, learning strategies, responsibility, and healthy-unhealthy behaviors, which was given by two specialists on educational psychology. They were also encouraged to contact the PE teacher in case they faced learning or discipline problems with their children, or to be informed about their children's progress.

Students were encouraged to discuss with their parents several topics they were taught in PE class (e.g., why a goal for learning and personal improvement is more important than a goal for outperforming others and high normative performance, how someone can lose weight combining exercise and diet, the effects of cigarette smoking on health, how an adolescent can remain a non-smoker, and the difficulty of quitting smoking). The parents' signature was required for some homework to ensure they were aware of their children's assiduity in their work. Furthermore, as described below, parents were "the sample" of a research project of students.

Improvement in the Health Domain

Intervention on goals in the health domain: Goal setting program to improve health indices. Students were asked to follow a personal goal-setting program to improve flexibility, strength, endurance, and body composition. Students kept their scores on flexibility, sit-up, shuttle run of speed tests of the Eurofit battery (Council of Europe, 1992), and body mass index (Wilcox, 1994). These scores were named health indices to reduce social evaluation concerns. The benefits of regular assessment of health indices were also pointed out. It was also stressed that these health indices should not be a point of comparison with others and that they would not be used for grading.

Students had a PE notebook where they kept their scores. After tests given in the beginning of the year and following an explanation of the goal setting procedure, students were asked to set a goal for personal improvement at 10-30% until the end of the term (three months later). Health indices were recorded again at the end of the second term.

Intervention on health outcomes: Promotion of exercise. As has been already described, students were encouraged to participate in sport activities at school in the afternoons, during school breaks, and on weekends with their parents.

Improvement in the Achievement Domain
Intervention on achievement goals:

(1) *Emphasis on personal improvement.* Through discussions and the goal setting program described below, the PE teachers emphasized the value of personal improvement in achievement domains such as PE, math, Greek language, and other academic subjects.

(2) *Reduction of competitive activities—promotion of cooperative activities.* Cooperative learning teaches students to be less egocentric and to respect the rights of others (Kirschenbaum, 1995). In our intervention few competitive activities, but a large number of cooperative activities, were used. Specific activities were applied, so that students would experience the positive effects of personal improvement goal orientation. Cooperation was emphasized in all kinds of activities, even in competitive games. For example, in a game of ball possession in basketball, points were awarded only if every player on the team managed to get a pass.

(3) *Inclusion.* All students had the chance to participate actively in the lesson. This philosophy of giving equal opportunities for success took place in all lessons, even those involving team games. For example, in soccer, boys and girls played together and a goal from a girl counted double points. These rules were introduced after a discussion with the students and upon their agreement. During practice, students were given the authority to choose training conditions by themselves, so as to succeed. For example, they could adapt the distance of shooting, and the number of trials, according to their personal needs.

Intervention on achievement outcomes:

(1) Increase of academic learning time. All lessons were carefully planned to sustain high levels of academic learning time (e.g., students were given task sheets and asked to exercise in groups of four to six to avoid long lines and wasting time).

(2) Reciprocal style of teaching. To increase cooperation, communication, and responsibility through the learning process, the reciprocal style of teaching was implemented in approximately 10% of the total teaching time (Moston & Asworth, 1994). Peers who acted as observers of their teammates' performance used performance criteria that were described on a task card given by the teacher. These students were particularly reminded to use positive feedback and avoid negative comments.

Teaching Interdisciplinary Skills

The present interdisciplinary teaching used tasks aiming at the development of self-regulation skills in sport, school, and life, and included projects connecting themes across sport and academic disciplines. Central to the intervention was a goal-setting program facilitating the adoption of personal improvement goals across a variety of human action domains and life contexts. A detailed description of this program is given by Milosis and Papaioannou (2007). Briefly, this program emphasized improvement goals and outcomes across contexts as follows.

Intervention on goals across contexts:

(1) Self-assessment and self-monitoring. First, students were helped to assess their records in health indices tests. Then, they applied self-assessment in other contexts, such as in math classes or in home activities requiring responsibility. For example, they were assessing the time needed to study, and using questionnaires, they assessed their level of respect toward others (Glazer, 1997; Nichols, & Utesch, 1998). Students were encouraged to monitor their progress and to print their scores on goal setting forms.

(2) Goal setting. Students were introduced to goal-setting in the beginning of the year. After a brief discussion about the meaning, the goal characteristics, and the method of application, the students were urged to practice the procedure. Students were asked to set long-term goals after graduation, then yearly goals for school and sport, and then more specific personal goals in PE, in other academic subjects (e.g., math, language) and in responsible behavior, and to commit themselves to their achievement. After being taught how to set challenging goals, the students were encouraged to set challenging goals in every PE class. Initially, students set goals to improve motor and psychological skills. Each lesson included at least one activity requiring the students to set either outcome or process goals (Zimmerman & Kitsantas, 1996). Gradually, this goal-setting program was expanded to the responsibility domain (e.g., make my bed every day), in core academic subjects (e.g., math, language) and in school in general (e.g., to spend 10 more minutes studying each subject or to solve one more math problem).

Gradually, the teacher transferred the responsibility of goal-setting to the students. For example, students were encouraged to select some goals on their own with the prompt, "decide by yourself," until they were gradually able to set their own goals. Moreover, in the second term, students chose specific skills from the health, achievement, and social domains in which they set monthly goals for personal improvement.

Intervention on outcomes across contexts:

(1) Psychological strategies such as positive self-talk, relaxation techniques, and positive thinking were used. Through the goal setting program, students were asked to use these strategies in other life settings, except for physical education, in both achievement and social domains.

(2) Learning strategies. Students were taught cognitive, metacognitive, and resource management strategies (Lapan, Kardash, & Turner, 2002; Weinstein & Mayer, 1986).

Promotion of Self-determination

Students were frequently asked to select activities, games, area, or equipment. They were encouraged to take responsibility for many of the auxiliary activities that facilitate sport participation, such as umpiring/

refereeing, coaching, and scorekeeping. Students were encouraged to participate actively in the modification of the rules, boundaries, and equipment of sporting activities, to enable everybody to find the lesson challenging (Hellison, 1995; Siedentop, 1994). In the second term, students were asked to cooperate in creating new games. They managed to create two new games with specific restrictions in terms of place, the number of players, and equipment. Through development of new games, students felt that they created something on their own, understood why rules are important and what purpose they serve, became involved in their own learning, shared their ideas and worked cooperatively, communicated and explained how their game developed, and taught others, including the teacher (Almond, 1986; Bunker & Thorpe, 1982).

Self-determination in the learning process was also promoted by asking students to use self-monitoring, by helping them to set goals and choose strategies based on the results of self-monitoring, and by using student-centered teaching styles such as the reciprocal, inclusion, self-check, discovery, and divergent styles (Mosston & Ashworth, 1994). These strategies offer experiences in respecting, trying, being self-directed, and caring (Hellison, 1996).

Organization

Organizational details of the intervention, such as the kind of assignments, assessment, class meetings, and structure of the class, are described in Milosis and Papaioannou (2007). These dimensions of teaching are important for the development of an adaptive motivational climate, the promotion of personal improvement goals, and the decrease of social evaluation in classes (Ames, 1992b). For example, self-assessment and peer-assessment were included in the evaluation process and were seriously considered by the teacher in assigning students' marks for the PE lesson; class meetings teach essential skills and empower young people with positive attitude for success in all areas of life: school, work, family, and society (Nelsen et al., 1997); and meaningful assignments are important components of the teaching process for the promotion of self-determination and personal improvement goals.

Results and Discussion

Based on results from confirmatory factor analyses, we established the structural validity of the global goal orientations questionnaire. For reasons of simplicity, these results are not reported here. As shown in Table 1 all scales were reliable.

To examine differences between experimental and control groups in the final measurements following adjustment of differences in the initial measurements, multivariate analyses of covariance (MANCOVAs) were conducted. Hence, covariates were the initial measurements, dependent variables were the final measurements, and independent variables the condition (experimental-control group). In all MANCOVAs significant main effects emerged.

As we expected, at the end of the intervention students in experimental classes had stronger personal improvement goals in life but lower ego-strengthening and ego-protection goals than students in control classes. Moreover, students in experimental classes had higher global self-determination, and specifically, higher intrinsic motivation and lower external regulation and amotivation than students in control classes. In addition, the intervention had positive effects on the general self-concept and the self-concept concerning honesty-trustworthiness. On the other hand, students in intervention classes had weaker intentions, perceived behavior control, and attitudes toward involvement in violent acts as fun.

To sum up, the adopted interdisciplinary program was effective in changing global psychological constructs such as goal orientations, self-determination, and self-concept. This is a very important finding because these global constructs affect adolescents' behaviors in all aspects of their life—not just in sport and school (see Williams, Cox, Hedberg, & Deci, 2000). Indeed, as the present intervention showed, the promotion of personal improvement goals in the responsibility domain was effective in terms of decreasing attitudes toward violence in sport-related events and increasing self-perceptions of honesty.

Elsewhere we have presented evidence suggesting that this intervention had substantial effects on achievement-related goals and self-perceptions in school and sport (Milosis & Papaioannou, 2007). Hence, the present interdisciplinary program had substantial effects on global goals, self-determination, and self-concepts,

Table 1. Scale Reliabilities and Results of the Final Measurements after
Multivariate Analyses of Covariance Controlling for the Initial Measurements

	Experimental group		Control group				
	M_{adj}	SE	M_{adj}	SE	F	Eta squared	Alpha
Goals in life							
Personal Development	4.50	.068	4.22	.050	5.83**	.04	.85
Ego-Strengthening	2.45	.088	3.02	.064	13.54***	.08	.79
Ego-Protection	2.43	.104	3.11	.076	21.20***	.12	.87
Social Approval	3.99	.095	3.85	.069	2.10	.01	.88
Global motivation							
Intrinsic Motivation	4.12	.071	3.91	.054	5.26**	.02	.88
Identified Regulation	3.91	.071	3.88	.054	.062	.00	.81
External Motivation	2.79	.094	3.39	.072	25.89***	.11	.77
Amotivation	2.20	.108	2.65	.082	11.15***	.05	.78
Self-Determination	4.92	.34	3.04	.26	18.66***	.08	-
Self-concept							
General Self	4.85	.066	4.45	.051	13.65***	.08	.75
Honesty-Trustworthiness	3.95	.089	3.74	.069	7.75***	.05	.79
Involvement in violent acts in sport-related events							
Attitudes	1.50	.153	2.14	.116	11.08***	.05	.95
Intentions	1.41	.149	1.97	.114	8.85**	.04	.96
Perceived Control	1.49	.146	1.89	.111	4.80*	.02	.95

Note: M = Estimated Marginal Means, controlling for initial differences before the intervention.

SE = Standard Error of the Mean.

Eta squared = Magnitude of Difference between the two Means. For eta squared higher than .15 the difference is considered large, between .06 and .14 the difference is considered moderate, less than .06 the difference is considered small.

Alpha = Cronbach's alpha reliability; when it is higher than .70 the scale is considered reliable.

*$p<.05$, **$p<.01$, ***$p<.001$

as well as on contextual goals and self-perceptions in sport and school concerning students' achievement and responsibility. Using an interdisciplinary program, we tried to affect goals, self-determination, self-perceptions, and their outcomes across various contexts (PE and sport, math, and language classes, in school in general, in the home, and with their peers), and through the accumulation of experiences in these contexts we reinforced their importance in life in general (i.e., at the global level of generality). We believe that the simultaneous effects on goal orientations at both global and contextual levels of generality strengthened the links between the two levels and facilitated the top-down and bottom-up effects. This boosted even further the effec-

tiveness of our program and the substantial effect sizes presented here and elsewhere (Milosis & Papaioannou, 2007) are supportive of this argument.

Our study benefited from the life skills programs adopted by leaders in this field (e.g., Danish, 1997; Gould, Collins, Lauer, & Chung, 2007). As in these studies, our students learned how to set goals for improvement in the physical activity setting, knowing what strategies to follow to achieve their goals and how to transfer these skills to other parts of their life. However, unlike studies that focused on life skills but not on goal orientations, we also focused on the motivational climate of classes. We did this because goals promoted by the environment affect students' willingness to adopt these skills in life. The selection of our tasks, our feedback, our assessment systems, and our student-centered approach were in line with theoretical propositions such as the TARGET model, which aims to develop a motivational climate promoting personal improvement goals and decreasing social evaluation and, correspondingly, performance goals (Papaioannou & Goudas, 1999; Treasure & Roberts, 1995). Hence, the life skills program was an essential part of an integrated intervention aimed at the promotion of personal development in life. Importantly, our focus on the personal improvement goals across contexts and in life in general boosted the meaningfulness of adopting life skills; it offered reasons why it is important to adopt these skills in life. The motto, "By pursuing personal improvement goals we will live a better life," was specified across settings primarily by the students themselves; for example, "By pursuing personal improvement goals in physical activity I will be healthier" or "By pursuing personal improvement goals in math I will...," etc.

To conclude, the present PE curriculum, based on the multidimensional model of goal orientations, adopted a holistic approach in the teaching process. Like others (e.g., Hellison & Templin, 1991; Zakrajsek & Carnes, 1986), this program emphasizes the holistic growth of the person, including physical, cognitive, emotional, and social development. We strongly believe that the adoption of this theoretical framework by PE teachers and coaches will enable them to provide substantial help to their students and athletes so that they will excel in sport, school, and life.

References

Ajzen, I. (1998). *Attitudes, personality and behaviour.* Bristol: Open University Press.

Almond, L. (1986). Games making. In R. Thorpe, D. Bunker, & L. Almond (Eds.), *Rethinking games teaching* (pp. 67-70). Loughborough, England: Department of Physical Education and Sport Science.

Ames, C. (1992a). Achievement goals and the classroom motivational climate. In D.H. Schunk & J. L. Meece (Eds.), *Student perceptions in the classroom* (pp. 327-348). Hillsdale, NJ: Lawrence Erlbaum Associates.

Ames, C. (1992b). Classrooms: Goals, structure, and student motivation. *Journal of Educational Psychology, 84,* 261-271.

Bandura, A. (1986). *Social foundations of thought and action: A social-cognitive theory.* Englewood Cliffs, NJ: Prentice Hall.

Bunker, D., & Thorpe, R. (1982). A model for the teaching of games in the secondary school. *Bulletin of Physical Education, 10,* 9-16.

Carver, C. S., & Scheier, M. F. (1998). *On the self-regulation of behavior.* Cambridge, UK: Cambridge University Press.

Commission for Fair Play (1990). *Fair play for kids.* Gloucester, ON: Author.

Conroy, D. E., Elliot, A. J., & Hofer, S. M. (2003). A 2 X 2 achievement goals questionnaire for sport: Evidence for factorial invariance, temporal stability, and external validity. *Journal of Sport and Exercise Psychology, 25,* 456-476.

Council of Europe (1992). *Eurofit-Eurotest for the assessment of physical fitness.* Strasbourg, France: Author.

Covington, M. V. (1992). *Making the grade: A self-worth perspective on motivation and school reform.* New York: Cambridge University Press.

Cox, R. H. (1994). *Sport psychology: Concepts and applications.* Madison, WI: Brown & Benchmark.

Danish S. J., & Donohue, T. (1995). Understanding media's influence on the development of antisocial and prosocial behavior. In R. Hampton, P. Jenkins, & T. Gullota (Eds.), *Preventing violence in America* (pp. 135-156). Thousand Oaks, CA: Sage.

Danish, S. J. (1997). Going for the goal: A life skills program for adolescents. In G. Albee & T. Gullota (Eds.), *Primary prevention works* (pp. 291-312). Thousand Oaks, CA: Sage.

Danish, S. J., & Nellen, V. C. (1997). New roles for sport psychologists: Teaching life skills through sport to at-risk youth. *Quest, 49,* 100-113.

Deci, E. L., & Ryan, R. M. (1985). *Intrinsic motivation and self-determination in human behaviour.* New York: Plenum.

Duda, J. L. (1989a). The relationship between task and ego orientation and the perceived purpose of sport among male and female high school athletes. *Journal of Sport and Exercise Psychology, 11,* 318-335.

Duda, J. L. (1989b). Goal perspectives, participation and persistence in sport. *International Journal of Sport Psychology, 20,* 42-56.

Duda, J. L. (2005). Motivation in sport: The relevance of competence and achievement goals. In A. J. Elliot & C. S. Dweck (Eds.), *Handbook of competence and motivation* (pp. 318-335). New York: Guilford.

Duda, J. L., & Nicholls, J. G. (1992). Dimensions of achievement motivation in schoolwork and sport. *Journal of Educational Psychology, 84,* 290-299.

Duda, J. L., Olson, L. K., & Templin, T. J. (1991). The relationship of task and ego orientation to sportsmanship attitudes and the perceived legitimacy of injurious acts. *Research Quarterly for Exercise & Sport, 62,* 79-87.

Elliot, A. J. (2005). A conceptual history of the achievement goal construct. In A. Elliot & C. Dweck (Eds.), *Handbook of competence and motivation* (pp. 52-72). New York: Guilford.

Gibbons, S., & Ebbeck, V. (1997). The effect of different teaching strategies on the moral development of physical education students. *Journal of Teaching in Physical Education, 17,* 85-98.

Glazer, S. M. (1997). To build self-esteem, know the self. *Teaching PreK-8, 27,* 102-103.

Gould, D., Collins, K., Lauer, L., & Chung, Y. (2006). Coaching life skills: A working model. *Sport and Exercise Psychology Review, 2,* 4-12.

Gould, D., Collins, K., Lauer, L., & Chung, Y. (2007). Coaching life skills through football: A study of award winning high school coaches. *Journal of Applied Sport Psychology, 19,* 16-37.

Greek Ministry of Education (2003). *The official gazette, 303/*13-03–2003. Athens, Greece: Author.

Guay, F., Blais, M. R., Vallerand, R. J., & Pelletier, L. G. (1996). *The global motivation scale.* Unpublished manuscript, Universite du Quebec a Montreal.

Guay, F., Mageau, G. A., & Vallerand, R. J. (2003). On the hierarchical structure of self-determined motivation: A test of top-down, bottom-up, reciprocal, and horizontal effects. *Personality and Social Psychology Bulletin, 29,* 992-1004.

Hellison, D. (1995). *Teaching responsibility through physical activity.* Champaign, IL: Human Kinetics.

Hellison, D. (1996). Teaching personal and social responsibility in physical education. In S. J. Silverman & C. D. Ennis (Eds.), *Student learning in physical education* (pp. 269-286). Champaign, IL: Human Kinetics.

Hellison, D. R., & Templin, T. J. (1991). *A reflective approach to teaching physical education.* Champaign, IL: Human Kinetics.

Kavussanu, M., & Ntoumanis, N. (2003). Participation in sport and moral functioning: Does ego-orientation mediate their relationship? *Journal of Sport & Exercise Psychology, 25,* 501-518.

Kavussanu, M., & Roberts, G. C. (2001). Moral functioning in sport: An achievement goal perspective. *Journal of Sport & Exercise Psychology, 23,* 37-54.

Kirschenbaum, H. (1995). *100 ways to enhance values and morality in school and youth settings.* Boston, MA: Allyn & Bacon.

Klieber, L., & Roberts, G. C. (1981). The effects of sport experience in the development of social character: An exploratory investigation. *Journal of Sport Psychology, 3,* 114-122.

Lapan, R. T., Kardash, C. M., & Turner, S. (2002). Empowering students to become self-regulated learners. *Professional School Counselling, 5,* 257-265.

Lickona, T. (1991). *Educating for character: How our schools can teach respect and responsibility.* New York: Bantam.

Lickona. T. (1997). Educating for character: A comprehensive approach. In A. Molnar (Ed.), *The construction of children's character.* Chicago: University of Chicago Press.

Marsh, H. W., & Yeung, A. S. (1998). Top-down, BU, and horizontal models: The direction of causality in multidimensional, hierarchical self-concept models. *Journal of Personality and Social Psychology, 75,* 749-761.

Marsh, H. W., Parker, J., & Barnes, J. (1985). Multidimensional adolescent self-concepts: Their relationship to age, sex, and academic measures. *American Educational Research Journal, 22,* 422-444.

Milosis, D., & Papaioannou, A. (2007). Interdisciplinary teaching, multiple goals and self-concept. In J. Liukkonen (Ed.), *Psychology for physical educators* (Vol. 2, pp. 175-198). Champaign, IL: Human Kinetics.

Morris, G. S. D. (2003). Social responsibility through physical activity. In A. Laker (Ed.), *The future of physical education: Building a new pedagogy* (pp. 54–81). London and New York: Routledge.

Mosston, M., & Ashworth, S. (1994). *Teaching physical education.* New York: Macmillan.

Nelsen, J., Lott, L., & Glenn, H. S. (1997). *Positive discipline in the classroom.* Roseville, CA: Prima Publishing.

Nicholls, J. G. (1989). *The competitive ethos and democratic education.* Cambridge, MA: Harvard University Press.

Nichols, J. D., & Utesch, W. E. (1998). An alternative learning program: Effects on student motivation and self-esteem. *Journal of Educational Research, 91,* 272-278.

Noddings, N. (1992). *The challenge to care in schools: An alternative approach to education.* New York: Teachers College Press.

Ntoumanis, N. (2001). Empirical links between achievement goal theory and self-determination theory in sport. *Journal of Sports Sciences, 19,* 397-409.

Ntoumanis, N., & Biddle, S. (1999). A review of motivational climate in physical activity. *Journal of Sports Sciences, 17,* 643–665.

Ommundsen, Y. (2003). Implicit theories of ability and self-regulation strategies in physical education classes. *Educational Psychology 23,* 141-157.

Papaioannou, A. (1998). Goal perspectives, reasons for being disciplined and self-reported discipline in the lesson of physical education. *Journal of Teaching in Physical Education, 17,* 421-441.

Papaioannou, A. (1999). Towards multidimensional hierarchical models of motivation in sport. *Proceedings of the 10th European Congress of Sport Psychology – FEPSAC* (Part 1, pp. 45-52). Prague: Charles University.

Papaioannou, A. (2006). Muslim and Orthodox Christian students' goal orientations at different levels of generality and life contexts. *International Journal of Sport & Exercise Psychology, 4,* 250-282.

Papaioannou, A., & Goudas, M. (1999). Motivational climate of the physical education class. In Y. Vanden Auweele, F. Bakker, S. Biddle, M. Durand, & R. Seiler (Eds.), *Psychology for physical educators* (pp. 51–68). Champaign, IL: Human Kinetics.

Papaioannou, A., Bebetsos, E., Theodorakis, Y., Christodoulidis, T., & Kouli, O. (2006). Causal relationships of sport and exercise involvement with goal orientations, perceived competence and intrinsic motivation in physical education: A longitudinal study. *Journal of Sports Sciences, 24,* 367-382.

Papaioannou, A., Karastogiannidou, C., & Theodorakis, Y. (2004). Sport involvement, sport violence and health behaviors of Greek adolescents. *European Journal of Public Health, 14,* 168-172.

Papaioannou, A., Milosis, D., Kosmidou E., & Tsigilis, N. (2002). Multidimensional structure of goal orientations: The importance of adopting a personal development goal in physical education. *Hellenic Journal of Psychology, 9,* 494-513.

Papaioannou, A., Tsigilis, N., Kosmidou, E., & Milosis, D. (2007). Measuring perceived motivational climate in physical education. *Journal of Teaching in Physical Education, 26,* 236-259.

Papaioannou, G. A., Ampatzoglou, G., Kalogiannis, P., & Sagovits, A. (in press). Social agents, achievement goals, satisfaction and academic achievement in youth sport. *Psychology of Sport & Exercise.*

Siedentop, D. (1994). *Sport education: Quality PE through positive sport experiences.* Champaign, IL: Human Kinetics.

Solmon, M. A., & Lee, A. M. (1997). Development of an instrument to assess cognitive processes in physical education classes. *Research Quarterly for Exercise and Sport, 68,* 152-160.

Standage, M., Duda, J. L., & Ntoumanis, N. A. (2003). Model of contextual motivation in physical education: Using constructs from self-determination and achievement goal theories to predict physical activity intentions. *Journal of Educational Psychology, 95,* 97-110.

Theodorakis, Y., Papaioannou, A., & Karastogiannidou, C. (2004). The relationship between family structure and students' health related attitudes and behaviors. *Psychological Reports, 95,* 851-858.

Theodosiou, A., & Papaioannou, A. (2006). Motivational climate, achievement goals, and metacognitive activity in physical education and exercise involvement in out-of-school settings. *Psychology of Sport & Exercise, 7,* 361-380.

Treasure, D., & Roberts, G. (1995). Applications of achievement goal theory to physical education: Implications for enhancing motivation. *Quest, 47,* 475-489.

Vallacher, R. R., & Wegner, D. M. (1987). What do people think they're doing? Action identification and human behavior. *Psychological Review, 94,* 3-15.

Vallerand, R. J. (1997). Toward a hierarchical model of intrinsic and extrinsic motivation. In M. P. Zanna (Ed.), *Advances in experimental social psychology* (pp. 271-360). New York: Academic Press.

Weinstein, C. E., & Mayer, R. E. (1986). The teaching of learning strategies. In M. Wittrock (Ed.), *Handbook of research on teaching* (pp. 315-327). New York: Macmillan.

Wilcox, K. L. (1994). BMI: *Improving its ability to predict body fat.* Master's Thesis, Brigham Young University, UK.

Williams, G. C., Cox, E. M., Hedberg, V. A., & Deci, E. L. (2000). Extrinsic life goals and health-risk behaviors in adolescents. *Journal of Applied Social Psychology, 30,* 1756-1771.

Zakrajsek, D., & Carnes, L. A. (1986). *Individualizing physical education.* Champaign, IL: Human Kinetics.

Zimmerman, B. J., & Kitsantas, A. (1996). Self-regulated learning of a motoric skill: The role of goal-setting and self-monitoring. *Journal of Applied Sport Psychology, 8,* 60-75.

CHAPTER 9

Research on Arab Sport Excellence

When examining the sport psychology literature, we note that the majority of the research published is restricted to a single ethnic group, which generally comes from North America and Europe. Therefore, it becomes difficult and unclear whether the results of these studies could be generalized to other populations, because few comparative and cross-cultural studies have appeared in the literature. Duda and Allison (1990), evoking the relevance of cross-cultural studies in sport, argued that sport in general cannot be understood if it is only observed in isolated ethnic environments. Although the call for more comparative and cross-cultural studies has been made by several researchers in sport psychology (e.g., Baria, 1987; Baria & Salmela, 1988; Cox, Yijun, & Zhan, 1993; Duda & Allison, 1990), this kind of inquiry remains rare in the Western world and neglected in the Arab sport literature, where the religious as well as cultural factors act as a powerful force. This study is intended to illuminate this issue.

This chapter is divided into two sections, and will deal with issues in Arab countries. In the first section, I will present a brief overview designed to compare the

evolution of Arab sport psychology to that of the Western world. The second section consists of the presentation of a study focused on the psychological ingredients for success and excellence in Arab sport (Baria & Nabli, 2001).

Evolution of Arab Sport Psychology

Over the last three decades sport psychology has experienced remarkable growth in Western countries. The number of sport psychologists and sport psychology societies, particularly in North America and Europe, is constantly increasing. However, in Arab countries this discipline is growing at a modest rate, because athletes, coaches, and sport administrators are only beginning to become aware of the important role that sport psychology and mental training play in sport excellence (Allawy, 2004; Baria & Salmela, 1987; Salmela, 1992). As indicated in *The World Sport Psychology Sourcebook* (Lidor, Morris, & Bardaxoglu, 2001; Salmela, 1992), Arab countries do not yet have an academic and professional program in sport psychology that has reached its

RESEARCH ON ARAB SPORT EXCELLENCE   91

full potential. Instead, the category of professionals we usually meet in the Arab countries are academicians, generally university professors, who are involved in the discovery of knowledge related to sport psychology, as well as its dissemination to sport actors such as athletes, coaches, sport managers, and parents. On the other hand, professionals who provide practical intervention services to athletes and coaches remain rare. This category of professionals is not yet well established and continues to be a deficit in the general training and programming of the Arab athletes. This fact is due to a lack of practical and applied education available to Arab sport psychologists, as well as to the skepticism of the persons in charge of sport regarding the benefits of mental training on performance.

In terms of sport psychology research, most of the studies conducted in the Arab countries have traditionally been descriptive and limited to theoretical psychological aspects. Research in this field is generally conducted by professors and faculties of physical education departments or by graduate students interested in the discipline. The topics that have received considerable attention are related to athletes' personality (Arfa, 2004; Ouadghiri, 1988), anxiety (Allawy, 1997, 2004), causal attribution (El Arabi & Esmail, 1987), motivation (Nabli, Baria, & Oubahammou, 2003a, b), and observation of the competitive behaviors of athletes (Baria, 1987, 2004; Baria & Salmela, 1988; El Arabi & Esmail, 1987). In general, these studies are basically not original or innovative; they generally expand on earlier findings and are predominantly influenced by the work of Western sport psychology researchers. The typical research model used in these studies compares successful and unsuccessful athletes of different ages, gender, and levels of performance. The instruments frequently employed are often based on the use of translated and validated psychological inventories coming from North America and Europe (for review see Allawy, 2004; Baria, Nabli, & Oubahammou, 2003; Nabli et al., 2003a, b).

In terms of applied sport psychology research, the low productivity rate of studies in this area remains a cause of concern in Arab countries, because the level of professional involvement with elite athletes is still modest. Therefore, the potential for development of applied sport psychology would be greater if there were a sufficient involvement accompanied by a political will from sport-related bodies, such as the Olympic committees, ministries of sport, and sport federations. Thus, as is

the case in the Western countries and some Asian countries (e.g., Russia, Japan, China, Korea, and Taiwan), to better prepare athletes psychologically and to foster the beneficial development of the field, Arab sport authorities are required to initiate efforts to provide sport psychology services to their respective national teams who participate in international competitions. In addition, they should support individuals who are interested in the domain to pursue clinical or counseling and sport psychology training. Lastly, in order to develop the applied sport psychology research in Arab countries, it is crucial to make a shift from the traditional descriptive research to an in-depth and idiographic research paradigm that examines and uncovers the real factors leading to athletic excellence.

Moroccan Elite Athletes' Views of Sport Excellence

As mentioned above, the second section of this chapter will focus on a particular research study my colleagues and I have conducted to investigate the perception of Moroccan elite athletes toward sport excellence. However, before presenting this study, it would be interesting to give a brief overview of research already done in this domain of interest. Over the last 15 years, a great deal of research has been carried out in the area of sport psychology in order to understand the reasons and conditions of emergence of high-level performance in sport. Two research paradigms have been used to examine psychological characteristics associated with athletic success. The first involves a quantitative methodology assessing the psychological abilities and elements of successful versus unsuccessful athletes via self-report instruments (e.g., Mahoney, Gabriel, & Perkins, 1987; for a review see Williams, 1986). Results of these quantitative investigations reveal that successful athletes are more self-confident, are better able to concentrate, are more committed and motivated, and are better able to cope with stress than their less successful counterparts. In one of the few studies in an Arab context examining the sources of success in sport, Baria et al. (2003) quantitatively assessed the perceptions of 546 Moroccan athletes of different ages and gender regarding the causes of success in sport. The subjects completed an Arabic-translated version of the Questionnaire of Perceived Causes of Success in Sport (QPCSS) elaborated upon by Duda and White (1992). Baria and his colleagues found that success is mutually assigned to internal factors such as effort and ability—factors that are under the individual's control. Moreover, male and female athletes seemed to be homogeneous in terms of their beliefs regarding the causes of sport success. The authors concluded that success in sport, as perceived by the Moroccan athletes, stems from a person's total commitment, hard work, fair play, and love of the training.

The second paradigm of sport psychology research relates to a qualitative approach, which is beginning to be considered as one of the best methods to inductively identify the main components of a knowledge domain. Orlick and Partington's (1988) "Mental Links to Excellence" investigation of Canadian elite athletes who participated in the 1984 Olympic Games in Sarajevo and Los Angeles has been at the forefront of qualitative studies designed to identify the mental components associated with athletic excellence. Based on results of various studies with world-class athletes as well as individuals engaged in other high-performance pursuits, Orlick (1992) formulated a conceptual Model of Human Excellence called the "Wheel of Excellence," that includes seven mental elements of excellence: commitment, confidence, full focus, positive imagery, mental readiness, distraction control, and ongoing learning. This model was used as a basic framework for the present study.

Since 1993 there has been another sort of research examining the origins of expertise and excellence in sport (see Ericsson, 1996; Ericsson, Krampe, & Römer, 1993; Starkes, Deakin, Allard, Hodges, & Hayes, 1996). These studies reveal that athletic expertise is primarily a result of practice and training, rather than innate talent or physical and physiological characteristics. These authors are unanimous in their belief that the level of skill has a positive linear relationship with the amount of accumulated practice throughout an athlete's sport career. Thus, according to Ericsson et al. (1993), what we call excellence in sport seems to be due to a biological adaptation that results from "deliberate practice." In spite of this, the Arab sport literature offers little information regarding issues which lead to expertise. According to these considerations, it would be interesting for sports administrators in Arab countries to revise their sport vision, which traditionally has been centered on the identification and selection of sport talents rather than on the practice and training to achieve sport excellence.

When examined collectively, these studies have provided interesting findings on the psychological aspects associated with athletic success. However, they have always been bound by Western standards. Consequently, because few comparative studies have appeared in the worldwide literature, it is not possible to generalize their results across Arab nations or other countries. It is within such a perspective that the present research was carried out. This idiographic study aims to gain a better understanding of what it takes for Moroccan elite athletes to be mentally successful in the highly competitive environment of elite sport. Indeed, from a comparative perspective, one can only speculate on whether athletes who grew up in a developing nation (e.g., Arab countries) with a specific cultural and religious background, and in which performance levels are limited because of financial or technical resources, would perceive the ingredients of sport excellence in a similar way to those of Western athletes.

The sample of the study included twenty of the most accomplished Moroccan athletes in track and field (two women Olympic athletes, three male record holders, two male Olympic athletes, and five high-level athletes), soccer (six professional male players), and tennis (two professional male players). Their sport experience varied from 9 to 18 years, which classified them as experts (Ericsson et al., 1993).

The subjects were interviewed using a combination of structured and unstructured questions to gain knowledge of their perceptions of the elements of sport excellence. The interviews started with general information being provided about the purpose of the project and then focused on gaining demographic information from the participants. The interviews were in the Arabic language. Each interview was tape-recorded with the permission of the respondent and then translated into English. The interview transcripts were inductively analyzed with the procedures outlined by Côté, Salmela, Baria, and Russell (1993). A software program for interpretational qualitative analysis helped in the analyses of the athletes' interviews. A selection of interview quotations illustrates the most important factors related to sport excellence.

Results of this study reveal that for Moroccan athletes, commitment and confidence appear to be the most important factors that allowed them to achieve the highest levels of excellence. They estimated that commitment and confidence are interdependent; as confidence and belief are strengthened, commitment is enhanced. The meaning-units presented throughout the results illustrate the importance of each component.

Commitment

For the athletes involved in this study, commitment constitutes an essential factor of excellence. All these athletes have insisted on the role that commitment plays in the realization of exceptional performance. Their commitment was evidenced by their dedication, sacrifice, willingness, perseverance, patience, and responsibility. The following quotes clearly illustrate how commitment was perceived by these athletes.

> In the beginning, it was a simple game. I practiced my sport with friends for the pleasure, but after that I worked hard to become professional. It is necessary to commit 100%, to work hard, to love this work and respect it. (Professional soccer player)

> To reach the goal, an athlete has to make sacrifices. For example, this year, I have spent most the time in Ifrane (a city in the Atlas Mountains), far from my parents and my friends, because this is the year of Olympic Games, and that counts a lot in my career as an athlete. (Olympic champion)

> For a woman athlete to reach the international level, she has to sacrifice several feminine aspects, among others, her hairstyle, her feminine figure, etc. She has to forget all the "coquette clothing" aspect. It means that Moroccan women athletes cannot access the international level without sacrifices. (Women's world champion)

> Because of my studies, I only practiced two times per week. I decided to abandon them and to devote myself to athletics, and then I began to practice two times per day in order to be a high-level athlete such as Nawal El Moutawakel. (Women's world champion)

Confidence

According to this factor, the results show that Moroccan elite athletes seem to maintain a high level of confidence. The analysis of the transcriptions of the different interviews shows that these athletes are essentially competitors with a tough mental attitude, which helps maintain their high level of confidence. They believe in their capacity to reach their goals, and remain trustful even in difficult situations. These characteristics are illustrated in the following quotations:

> The material conditions are not very important; it all depends on the individual and on his conviction for success... Thinking about the record of Saîd Aouita that lasted 8 years, I said to myself it is necessary that a Moroccan beats this record; I made it because I was determined and I had will. I could improve while working harder to achieve a goal; it is necessary to have confidence and belief that you can reach it. (Olympic champion and record holder)

> I had self-confidence. I told myself: good, I am in good physical and mental shape, I have trained the best I can, and then I have to win. (International athlete)

Some Moroccan athletes regard as very important the establishment of a climate of mutual confidence between the athlete and the environment. This climate translates into the confidence that athletes have in their coach or the conviction that other people have in their capacity to achieve excellence. These external elements of confidence are expressed in the following meaning units:

> As an elite athlete, you know what you are capable of; you have confidence in your ability. But, this is not sufficient; you need the confidence of other persons such as your coach, your parents, and your friends about your potential, and they should incite you to resist. (Professional tennis player)

> The athlete must have confidence in his coach, since he plans his training and determines the volume and the intensity of work. Without confidence, you cannot go far; you can find any pretext to avoid the practice. (International athlete)

Concentration

The major performance blocks that interfered with Moroccan elite athletes were concentration, distraction control, and ongoing learning. When interviewed, few athletes mentioned the importance of concentration in training. A large number of them mentioned that they had not yet learned how to focus better when distractions haunt them. However, as expressed by the quotations below, some of these athletes had developed their own strategies, such as praying or reading the Koran, to better concentrate. Their confessions seem to give them moral support to overcome situations that can affect their performance.

> Frankly I have not learned how to concentrate. But, ten minutes before the competition, I avoid speaking to anybody, I want to concentrate alone. I see myself on a beach, I read some verses of Koran and I repeat them until the start. After this, all my attention is focused on the tactics of my opponents. (Record holder)

> To concentrate before the competition, most Moroccan athletes make their prayers and repeat Koran verses before the start of the race; it is a type of concentration. (International record holder)

> I made a good start. I was so totally concentrated that I did not hear the noises of spectators. I try to concentrate solely on my race. (Olympic women's champion)

> When I meet my opponents in a training place, I repeat the following expression to encourage myself: "I am the strongest." I repeat this expression three or four times. It allows me to be combative and therefore to avoid thinking that I am the weakest among these athletes. This strategy allows me to be tough and have a good focus. (Olympic women's champion)

Distraction Control

Distractions before competition seem to present a potential performance block to Moroccan elite athletes. In the following quotations, some athletes relate their lack of ability to manage the distraction factors generated by the competition and by the national staff.

> You should have the quality to exclude all factors that could distract your mind and your vision, such as spectators, opponent, media, etc. I knew that every time I began to think about them, I would lose my concentration and my control. I'm aware of that, so all I had to do and think was: relax, laugh, and take it easy. (Professional tennis player)

> Everybody predicted that I would win a gold medal—the public, the press, the national staff, and the trainers, and yet I could not achieve their expectations. Indeed, I was very stressed and I felt the pressure of all these people, which I thought was the cause of my bad performance. (International athlete)

Positive Images (Imagery)

The results of the present survey show that some of the Moroccan athletes are aware of the importance of mental imagery to achieve excellence in sport. This strategy helps them to repeat the race or the skills in their minds so that they will be ready for the competition.

> In reality, I play the game three times, the real match plus two others in my mind (before and after the match). Before the match, I imagine how I am going to play, how to apply the instructions of the coach and the strategies recommended for the match. After the match, I visualize the movie in my head. (Professional soccer player)

> The athlete has to run the race in his head and has to imagine the strategies that he can adopt at the time of the race. (International athlete)

When interviewed, few Moroccan athletes considered ongoing learning and constructive evaluation as a prerequisite for their preparation. When they set their short- and long-term goals, they don't assess them and tend to neglect the evaluation of their performances. They justify this behavior by saying that they do not have the time or any theoretical knowledge for evaluation.

Conclusions

The findings of the present study clearly indicate that Moroccan elite athletes associate several mental elements with excellence in sport. For these athletes commitment, confidence, distraction control, and positive images seem to be the major factors that determine their success. Otherwise, and in contrast to the Western athletes interviewed by Orlick and Partington (1988), they don't seem to value mental readiness and ongoing learning. This led us to believe that to achieve their potential, Moroccan athletes should become more aware of the importance of the elements that constitute the Orlick "Wheel of Excellence."

This study aimed to convey new information on the field of Arab sport excellence. It provides Arab coaches, athletes, and sport administrators with a portrait of how top Arab athletes perceive the elements that lead to sport excellence and how they have climbed the ladder of excellence to reach the top.

References

Allawy, H. M. (1997). *Sport psychology.* Cairo, Egypt: Centre d'édition.

Allawy, H. M. (2004). The development of sport psychology in Egypt. In A. Baria & H. Nabli (Eds.), *Introduction of sport psychology in Africa: 1st International Congress of Sport Psychology* (pp. 250-255). Marrakech, Morocco.

Arfa, Y. (2004). Les traits de personalité comme determinants des marges de développement des capacités physiques chez les joueurs de handball. In A. Baria & H. Nabli (Eds.), *Introduction of sport psychology in Africa: 1st International Congress of Sport Psychology* (pp. 69-81). Marrakech, Morocco.

Baria, A. (1987). *Les comportements individuels et interpersonnels pre et post-performance des gymnastes arabes.* Unpublished master's thesis, University of Montréal, Montréal, Québec.

Baria, A. (1994). *Une analyse comparative des perceptions des entraineurs internationaux à l'égard des connaissances reliées au processus de coaching en gymnastique.* Unpublished doctoral thesis, University of Ottawa, Ottawa, Canada.

Baria, A., & Nabli, H. (2001). Sport psychology in Morocco. In R. Lidor, T. Morris, E. Bardaxoglu, & B. Becker (Eds.), *The world sport psychology sourcebook* (3rd ed., pp. 30-32). Morgantown, WV: Fitness Information Technology.

Baria, A., Nabli, H., & Oubahammou, L. (2003). Perceptions about the causes of sport success among Moroccan athletes and coaches. In R. Stelter (Ed.), *New approaches to exercise and sport psychology: Theory, methods and applications.* Eleventh European Congress of Sport Psychology, Copenhagen, Denmark.

Baria, A., & Salmela, J. H. (1987). Comportements post-compétitifs des gymnastes Arabes. In J. H. Salmela, B. Petiot, & T. B. Hoshisaki (Eds.), *Psychological nurturing and guidance of gymnastic talent* (pp. 149-162). Montréal: Sport Psyche.

Baria, A., & Salmela, J. H. (1988). Competitive behaviors of Arabic and Olympic gymnasts. *International Journal of Sport Psychology, 3,* 171-183.

Côté, J., Salmela,, J. H., Baria, A., & Russell, S. J. (1993). Organizing and interpreting unstructured qualitative data. *The Sport Psychologist, 7,* 127-137.

Cox, H. R., Yijun, Q., & Zhan L. (1993). Overview of sport psychology. In R. N. Singer, M. Murphy, & K. Tennant (Eds.), *Handbook of research on sport psychology* (pp. 3-31). New York: Macmillan.

Duda, J. L., & Allison, M. T. (1990). Cross-cultural analysis in exercise and sport psychology: A void in the field. *Journal of Sport & Exercise Psychology, 12,* 114-131.

Duda, J. L., & White, S. A. (1992). Goal orientation and beliefs about the causes of sport success among elite skiers. *The Sport Psychologist, 6,* 334-343.

El Arabi, M., & Esmail, M. (1987). Competitive behaviors of Egyptian gymnasts. In J. H. Salmela, B. Petiot, & T. B. Hoshisaki (Eds.), *Psychological nurturing and guidance of gymnastic talent* (pp. 149-162). Montréal: Sport Psyche.

Ericsson, K. A. (1996). The acquisition of the expert performance: An introduction to some of the issues. In K. A. Ericsson (Ed.), *The road to excellence: The acquisition of the expert performance in the art and sciences, sports and games* (pp. 1-50). Mahwah, NJ: Erlbaum.

Ericsson, K. A., Krampe, R. T., & Römer, C. T. (1993). The role of deliberate practice in the acquisition of expert performance. *Psychological Review, 3,* 363-406.

Lidor, R., Morris, T., Bardaxoglu, E., & Becker, B. (2001). *The world sport psychology sourcebook* (3rd ed.). Morgantown, WV: Fitness Information Technology.

Mahoney, M. J., Gabriel, T. J., & Perkins, R. S. (1987). Psychological skills and exceptional athletic performance. *The Sport Psychologist, 1,* 181-199.

Nabli, H., Baria, A., & Oubahammou, L. (2003a). An international and comparative study of motivation profiles among scholar cross-country athletes. In R. Stelter (Ed.), *New approches to exercise and sport psychology: Theory, methods and applications.* Eleventh European Congress of Sport Psychology, Copenhagen, Denmark.

Nabli, H., & Baria, A., & Oubahammou, L. (2003b). Motivation profiles of Moroccan athletes. In R. Stelter (Ed.), *New approches to exercise and sport psychology: Theory, methods and applications.* Eleventh European Congress of Sport Psychology, Copenhagen, Denmark.

Orlick, T. (1992). The psychology of personal excellence. *Contemporary Thought on Performance Enhancement, 1,* 109-122.

Orlick, T., & Partington, J. (1988). Mental links to excellence. *The Sport Psychologist, 2,* 105-130.

Ouadghiri, K. (1988). *La personnalité des joueurs marocains de football. Mémoire de fin d'études.* Rabat, Maroc: Institut National des Sport.

Salmela, J. H. (1992). *The world sport psychology sourcebook.* Champaign, IL: Human Kinetics.

Starkes, J. L., Deakin, J., Allard, F. Hodges, N. J., & Hayes, A. (1996). Deliberate practice in sports: What is it anyway? in K. A. Ericsson (Ed.), *The road to excellence: The acquisition of the expert performance in the art and sciences, sports and games* (pp. 81-106). Mahwah, NJ: Erlbaum.

Williams, J. M. (1986). Psychology characteristics of peak performance. In J. M. Williams (Ed.), *Applied sport psychology: Personal growth to peak performance* (pp. 123-132). Palo Alto, CA: Mayfield.

CHAPTER 10

The Road to Continued Sport Participation and Sport Excellence

JEAN CÔTÉ

An athlete's sport performance during childhood is not a strong indicator of performance level in adulthood. In a review of the talent detection and development in sport literature, Régnier, Salmela, and Russell (1993) concluded that long-term prediction of talented athletes is unreliable, especially when detection of talent is attempted during the prepubertal or pubertal periods of growth. Côté and colleagues (Baker & Côté, 2006; Côté, Baker, & Abernethy, 2003, 2007) suggested that the most economical way of producing talent in sport is to provide sport programs from ages 6 to 12 that focus on children's needs and not on a rigid skill-based model. Sport programs that focus on play and children's development have been shown to lead to less dropout (Fraser-Thomas, Côté, & Deakin, 2008a, 2008b; Wall & Côté, 2007), continued participation in sport (Robertson-Wilson, Baker, Derbyshire, & Côté, 2003), and elite performance in adulthood (Baker, Côté, & Abernethy, 2003; Baker, Côté, & Deakin, 2005). On the other hand, children's sport programs that focus on a rigid skill-based

model imply an early selection of "talented" children, an increase in resources for a special group of athletes, and training that is not always consistent with the children's motivation to participate in sports. As such, some youth sport programs are designed with the long-term objective of producing elite-level athletes instead of serving the short-term needs of children.

In a review of the motor learning literature, Wulf and Shea (2002) distinguished between learning *effectiveness* and learning *efficiency*, both important issues in the study of complex motor skills and the development of expert performance in sport. Learning effectiveness focuses on factors that influence the acquisition of motor skills, while learning efficiency focuses on the factors that influence the acquisition of motor skills at less cost (Wulf & Shea, 2000). Learning efficiency considers the psychosocial (i.e., dropout) and physical (i.e., injury) costs associated with training and the development of expertise in sport. An *efficient* model of sport expertise development would limit the costs associated with long-term investment in sport, while an *effective* model would focus on learning independent of the costs that may be involved.

The *coefficient of efficiency* is the equivalent of an input-output ratio expressed as a percentage of the actual number of children that participate in a specific sport program at a given time (e.g., at age 10) over the number of the same children that participate in the same sport at a later time (e.g., at age 13). The coefficient of efficiency could be used as an indicator of the internal efficiency of a sport program for children (ages 6-12). The coefficient of efficiency could also be used as a measure of the quality of a childhood sport program by accounting for the dropout rate in the same sport from childhood to adolescence. A coefficient of efficiency of less than 100% from childhood sport participation to adolescence sport participation would indicate that certain children drop out of a specific sport and are no longer available to train for elite performance in this sport. Considering that performance in a given sport in childhood is a poor predictor of adult performance (Régnier et al., 1993), it is important that sport programs in childhood focus on retaining athletes by focusing on their level of efficiency. Sport programs with a strict emphasis on early selection, skill acquisition, and training during childhood might reduce their coefficient of efficiency and eliminate someone who, through growth, maturation, and training, later would develop into an elite-level athlete. The underpinning principle of highly *efficient* sport programs for childhood is to provide space, playing and training opportunities, and equipment for a large number of children across various sports. The framework of deliberate practice developed by Ericsson and colleagues, (Ericsson, 2003; Ericsson, Krampe, & Tesch-Römer, 1993) is an example of a model that is based on learning effectiveness during childhood, and accordingly, would receive a low coefficient of efficiency score. In their writing, Ericsson and colleagues suggest that it would be next to impossible for a late starter to overcome the early advantage gained by those who begin deliberate practice at a young age and maintain high amounts of deliberate practice hours over time. In sum, the framework of deliberate practice focuses on learning effectiveness, largely downplaying the psycho-social and physical costs associated with this type of practice, especially in the early years of an athlete's involvement in sport. While the positive relationship between training and elite performance is consistent in sport research

(Helsen, Starkes, & Hodges, 1998; Hodge & Deakin, 1998; Hodges & Starkes, 1996; Starkes, Deakin, Allard, Hodges, & Hayes 1996), few studies have analyzed the efficiency of sport programs that focus on a high amount of deliberate practice during childhood. Some data indicate that young elite ice hockey players who eventually dropped out began off-ice training (for the purpose of improving hockey performance) at a younger age and invested significantly more hours per year in off-ice training at ages 12-13 than a group of young elite ice hockey players who did not drop out (Wall & Côté, 2007). These results, along with qualitative data of dropout and burnout athletes (e.g., Carlson, 1988; Gould, Udry, Tuffey, & Loehr, 1996), indicate that sport programs that focus on high amounts of deliberate practice during childhood may receive a lower *coefficient of efficacy* rating than childhood sport programs that focus on play. Furthermore, intense and repeated training in one sport at a young age has been associated with higher rates of injuries (Brenner, 2007), which ultimately has an effect on the dropout rates of young athletes.

One model that focuses on learning efficacy and highlights the importance of developmentally appropriate training patterns and social influences is Côté and colleagues' Developmental Model of Sport Participation (DMSP; Figure 1; Côté, 1999; Côté et al., 2003, 2007; Côté & Fraser-Thomas, 2007; Côté & Hay, 2002). The DMSP proposed three sport participation trajectories: (1) recreational participation through sampling and deliberate play; (2) elite performance through sampling and deliberate play; and (3) elite performance through early specialization and deliberate practice. The different stages within a trajectory are based on changes in the type and amount of involvement in sport, play, and practice. Trajectories 1 and 2 imply a context of childhood sport participation that is characterized by a high amount of play and involvement in more than one sport through seasonal sport participation. The most important aspect of play and sampling in this context resides in the potential contribution of these activities in stimulating children's motivation to stay involved in sport.

Trajectory 1: Recreational Participation through Sampling and Deliberate Play

During the sampling years (age 6-12), athletes participate in a variety of sports with the focus being primarily on deliberate play activities. Deliberate play activities, such as "street hockey" or "backyard soccer,"

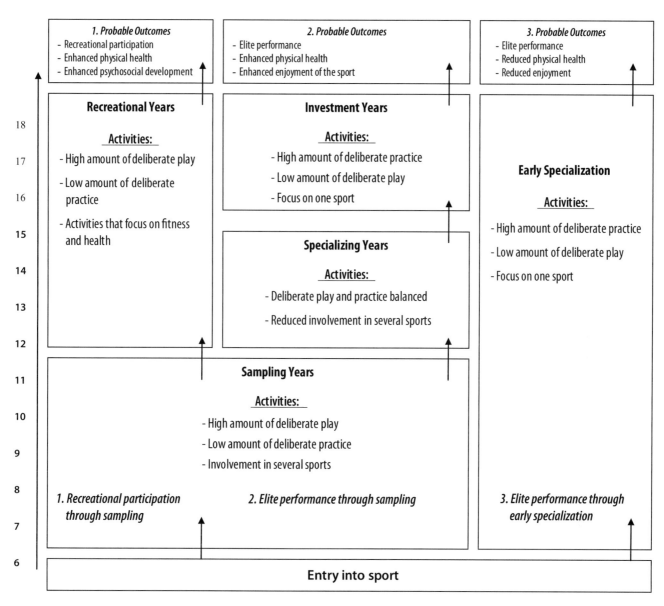

Figure 1. The developmental model of sport participation. Adapted from Côté, J., Baker, J., & Abernethy, B. (2007). Practice and play in the development of sport expertise. In R. Eklund & G. Tenenbaum (Eds.), *Handbook of sport psychology* (3rd ed., pp. 184-202). Hoboken, NJ: Wiley.

are regulated by flexible age-adapted rules, and are set up and monitored by children or an involved adult. The informality of deliberate play allows children to play sports with minimal equipment, in any kind of space, with any number of players, and with players of different ages and sizes (Côté et al., 2007). This kind of environment is easily created and does not require adult supervision, coaches, officials, specialized equipment, time limits, or uniforms that are characteristic of orga-

nized sport and structured practice. Through sampling various sports and engaging in deliberate play, the sampling years are considered essential building blocks for recreational sport participation and elite performance.

The recreational years (age 13+) are usually seen as an extension of the sampling years, with the primary goals being enjoyment and health. Activities can involve play and practice, and sport programs should be flexible enough to adapt to individual interests and ages.

Trajectory 2: Elite Performance through Sampling and Deliberate Play

For youth interested in a more performance-oriented path, a second trajectory of the DMSP recommends that specialization begin around age 13. After the sampling years, sport participants can embark on a path that focuses primarily on performance (*specializing years,* age 13-15; *investment years,* age 16+). Elite athletes who went through a stage such as the sampling years in their early involvement in sport tend to experience positive physical and psychosocial outcomes (e.g., physical health, sport enjoyment; Bloom, 1985; Carlson, 1988; Côté, 1999). In terms of producing elite-level performance, the specializing years (age 13-15) are seen as a transitional stage to the investment years (age 16+). During the specializing years, youth engage in fewer activities, which include both play and practice, while during the investment years, youth commit to only one activity, and engage primarily in practice. This trajectory toward elite performance in sport has been supported by various qualitative and quantitative studies (e.g., Baker et al., 2003, 2005; Carlson, 1988; Côté, 1999; Soberlak & Côté, 2003) and can be qualified as an *efficient* pathway to elite performance.

Trajectory 3: Elite Performance through Early Specialization and Deliberate Practice

A third trajectory to sport participation is elite performance through early specialization, which could be characterized as the most effective way to develop elite performance. Several studies support early specialization as a suitable path toward elite performance (see Ward, Hodges, Williams, & Starkes, 2004 for a review). Ericsson et al. (1993) defined deliberate practice as any training activity that (a) is undertaken with the specific purpose of increasing performance (e.g., not for enjoyment or external rewards), (b) requires cognitive and/or physical effort, and (c) is relevant to promoting positive skill development. Although studies in sport may support the fact that deliberate practice activities can result in pleasure or enjoyment (Starkes, 2000), deliberate practice activities are generally defined as being extrinsically motivated, literal, focused on outcomes rather than processes, and having somewhat rigid rules. Ericsson et al. (1993) suggested that "...the higher level of attained elite performance, the earlier the age of first exposure as well as the age of starting deliberate practice" (p. 389). The deliberate practice framework is therefore

in line with an early specialization pathway to elite performance. Elite performers that specialize at an early age usually skip the sampling years, and consequently, do not always experience the enjoyment associated with sampling and playing (Law, Côté, & Ericsson, 2007).

Few studies up to now have examined the dropout cost associated with early specialization in one sport and deliberate practice; however, dropout and injury studies suggest that sport programs adopting this philosophy may receive a coefficient of efficacy rating lower than sport programs that focus on children's play and sampling (i.e., Trajectories 1 and 2). In fact, there is reasonable empirical support for the notion that early specialization is associated with higher levels of attrition at all levels of ability (Fraser-Thomas et al., 2008a; Gould, 1987; Gould et al., 1996; Wall & Côté, 2007). Furthermore, an early focus on structured training can have negative effects on young athletes' physical health (Brenner, 2007; Caine, Cochrane, Caine, & Zemper, 1989).

Efficiency of Two Pathways To Elite Performance

Enough evidence exists to suggest two different pathways to elite performance in sport when peak performance is achieved after puberty (e.g., basketball, soccer, rowing, and triathlon). The main difference between the two pathways resides in the type of activities that children experience during their introduction to sport from ages 6 to 12. A first pathway suggested by Côté and colleagues (Côté et al., 2007; Côté & Fraser-Thomas, 2007) proposes that children's participation in deliberate play and seasonal sports are key elements for continued participation and investment in sport. A second pathway suggested by Ericsson and colleagues (Ericsson, 2003; Ericsson et al., 1993) proposes that deliberate practice and year-round participation in one sport is the best way to develop sport specific skills during childhood that are essential for adult elite performance in the same sport. Although no dropout rate figures exist for these two different pathways, it is possible to suggest a coefficient of efficiency that would be typical of these two different trajectories toward elite performance.

These two pathways can be hypothetically represented by two basketball programs for children (age 10). Each program is composed of 10 teams with 10 children per team for a total of 100 athletes per program. Program one, titled "Play," adheres to a philosophy of play and sampling and has children involved in basketball for a period of 4 months for 2 hours a week. The ratio of deliberate play/deliberate practice is approximately 80:20 in this program. In other words, every week children are involved in about 95 minutes of play-like activities and about 25 minutes of deliberate practice-like activities. Children in this program are also involved in at least three other sports throughout the year and have time to regularly play sports informally with their peers (i.e., deliberate play). Overall, children in this situation are involved in formal or informal sports for approximately 500 hours a year.

Program 2, titled "Practice," adheres to a deliberate practice philosophy and has children involved in basketball training year-round for approximately 10 hours per week. The ratio of deliberate play/deliberate practice is approximately 20:80 in this program. Every week children are involved in about 2 hours of deliberate play-like activity and 9 hours of deliberate practice. Children are discouraged from participating in other sports because of injury risk and are provided with an individualized training program, which, if followed, will increase their conditioning and possibly their future success in basketball. Therefore, it is strongly recommended by coaches and parents that children in this program spend their free time doing extra training. Like the 10-year-old children in the *Play* program, children in the *Practice* program are involved in approximately 500 hours per year in sport; however, their participation in sport is focused solely on basketball.

Based on these two scenarios, it is possible to forecast a rate of dropout for both programs, and accordingly suggest a coefficient of efficacy for each program. Empirical evidence strongly suggests that the *Practice* program is associated with higher levels of dropout in youth sport (Carlson, 1988; Fraser-Thomas et al., 2008a, 2008b; Gould, 1987; Gould et al., 1996; Wall & Côté, 2006). Although it is difficult to forecast an exact rate of dropout for each program, we can expect a higher dropout rate for the *Practice* program. Because of its focus on training and skill acquisition, the *Practice* program is more likely to lose children due to their lack of enjoyment, overtraining, injuries, burnout, stress, and anxiety (Butcher, Lindner, & Johns, 2002). Children commonly get involved in sport because "it's fun" (Brustad, Babkes, & Smith, 2001; Gould & Petlichkoff, 1988), while dropping out of sport includes more diverse reasons such as "interest in other activities," "lack of fun," "lack of playing time," "too little success," "loss of motivation," "dislike of the coach," "overemphasis on competition and performance," and "hard physical training" (Gould, 1987; Gould, Feltz, Horn, & Weiss, 1982; Orlick & Botterill, 1975). In sum, the "fun" aspect of sport appears to be the main reason for children's involvement (main emphasis of the *Play* program), while the competitive and more structured dimensions of sport are the catalyst for withdrawal (main emphasis of the *Practice* program).

If we suggest a dropout rate of 20% for the *Play* program, we can forecast a dropout rate of about 40% for the *Practice* program, because of additional dropout reasons such as "did not enjoy," "too much pressure to perform well," and "injury played a role," that would be unlikely in a *Play* program (Orlick & Botterill, 1975). Although youth sport programming in several countries is moving toward the implementation of *Practice*-like programs in children's sport, (Hecimovich, 2004; Hill, 1988; Hill & Hansen, 1988), recent developmental studies of dropout athletes suggest that environments that promote early specialization and deliberate practice in children's youth sport programs (such as the *Practice* program described above) lead to more dropout (Fraser-Thomas et al., 2008a, 2008b; Wall & Côté, 2007). Ultimately, at age 13, the *Play* program could have developed 80 children that love basketball but are not the most skilled players, and the *Practice* program could have developed 60 skilled basketball players that invest a large number of hours in basketball but may lack the commitment to pursue further training due to burnout symptoms (Raedeke, 1997; Raedeke & Smith, 2001).

Ideally, sport programs for children should aim at increasing their efficiency by reducing dropout instead of focusing on early selection, deliberate practice, and differentiation by children's skill abilities. From the hypothetical example described above, between the ages of 10 and 13, dropout averaging 40% in a *Practice* program results in a coefficient of efficiency of 60%. This implies that, on average, 40% of resources are wasted in this type of program and the chance of developing elite athletes is not necessarily greater. While it is impossible to completely eliminate dropout in children's sport, it is possible to create an environment (e.g., equal opportunities, fun) and provide activities (i.e., deliberate play and sampling) that are known to sustain children's commitment to stay in sport at both recreational and elite levels.

Support for an Elite Performance through Sampling Trajectory: The Birthplace Effect

A recent study by Côté, MacDonald, Baker, and Abernethy (2006) provides strong support for an *elite performance through sampling* trajectory that includes various types of sport involvement and play activities at a young age. An analysis of the birthplace of 2,240 professional athletes in basketball, baseball, ice hockey, and golf by Côté et al. showed a birthplace bias toward smaller cities, with professional athletes being overrepresented in cities of less than 500,000 and underrepresented in cities of 500,000 and more. The birthplace effect has recently been replicated in women's professional soccer and golf (King, MacDonald, Côté, & Abernethy, in press).

This birthplace effect has a significant influence on how athletes will first be exposed to sports, and can ultimately limit or benefit sport performance. For example, it is apparent that many children who live in smaller cities have access to resources that introduce them to sport in different ways than children from large urban areas. Urban athletes are more likely to practice their sport in a structured setting that resembles the *Practice* program described above. Such organized sport programs are built upon the principle of learning effectiveness and require a high level of human resources such as parental involvement, adult supervision, and coaching. Children's sport programs in bigger cities are more likely to focus on a rigid skill-based model (i.e., deliberate practice), imply an early selection of "talented" children, have increased resources for a special group of athletes, and consist of training that is not always consistent with the children's motivation to participate in sports. These models could be effective in sports where many children are available to compete, such as in bigger cities, and the cost of eliminating children has little effect on the overall goal of developing talent. On the other hand, children in smaller cities get involved in sport programs that are less selective and more inclusive because of the smaller number of children available to play sport. Sport programs in smaller cities are more likely to resemble the *Play* program described above, putting less emphasis on early acquisition of skills and performance and more emphasis on play and sampling. In other words, by putting an emphasis on learning efficiency instead of learning effectiveness, smaller cities may present more opportunities for the type of developmental experiences that characterize elite performance through the sampling trajectory of the DMSP.

Conclusion

Kirk (2005) discussed the impact of early learning experiences, competency, and skill development on young people's later involvement in sport. Drawing on the existing evidence about the psycho-social factors known to be important in children's learning of motor skills, Kirk proposed that sampling and deliberate play activities at a young age create an environment that increases children's exposure to sport and facilitates lifelong sport participation and expertise. Nevertheless, it appears that current trends in sport programming are moving toward institutionalization, elitism, early selection, and early specialization (Hecimovich, 2004; Hill, 1988; Hill & Hansen, 1988). Many sport programs are requiring higher levels of investment at earlier ages, and discourage children from participating in a diversity of activities (Gould & Carson, 2004; Hecimovich, 2004; Hill, 1988; Hill & Hansen, 1988). However, there is clear evidence suggesting that sport programs such as these may not be providing youths with optimal environments for lifelong involvement in sport and elite performance.

Overall, the different trajectories of the DMSP provide a useful framework for assessing the learning environments that lead to various performance and developmental outcomes in children. Although not all the outcomes of the DMSP have been directly tested, enough support exists to suggest developmental patterns that can be further tested through retrospective research. By considering factors other than accumulated amount of practice, the DMSP allows researchers to address questions regarding learning efficiency and learning effectiveness. A youth sport framework that focuses on learning efficiency should consider the various pathways that children follow in sport. Concerted effort is required from physical education teachers, coaches, and parents to ensure that children learn skills that will allow them to continue their participation in sport at either a recreational or an elite level.

References

Baker, J., & Côté J. (2006). Shifting training requirements during athlete development: The relationship among deliberate practice, deliberate play, and other sport involvement in the acquisition of sport expertise. In D. Hackfort & G. Tenenbaum (Eds.), *Essential processes for attaining peak performance* (pp. 93-110). Oxford, UK: Meyer and Meyer.

Baker, J., Côté , J., & Abernethy, B. (2003). Sport specific training, deliberate practice, and the development of expertise in team ball sports. *Journal of Applied Sport Psychology, 15,* 12-25.

Baker, J., Côté , J., & Deakin, J. (2005). Expertise in ultra-endurance triathletes: Early sport involvement, training structure, and the theory of deliberate practice. *Journal of Applied Sport Psychology, 17,* 64-78.

Bloom, B. S. (Ed.). (1985). *Developing talent in young people.* New York: Ballantine.

Brenner, J. S. (2007). Overuse injuries, overtraining, and burnout in child and adolescent athletes. *Pediatrics, 119,* 1242-1245.

Brustad, R. J., Babkes, M. L., & Smith, A. L. (2001). Youth in sport: Psychological considerations. In R. N. Singer, H. A. Hausenblas, & C. M. Janelle (Eds.), *Handbook of sport psychology* (2nd ed., pp. 604-635). New York: Wiley.

Butcher, J., Lindner, K. J., & Johns, D. P. (2002). Withdrawal from competitive youth sport: A retrospective ten-year study. *Journal of Sport Behavior, 25,* 145-163.

Caine, D., Cochrane, B., Caine, C., & Zemper, E. (1989). An epidemiologic investigation of injuries affecting young competitive female gymnasts. *American Journal of Sports Medicine, 17,* 811-820.

Carlson, R. C. (1988). The socialization of elite tennis players in Sweden: An analysis of the players' backgrounds and development. *Sociology of Sport Journal, 5,* 241-256.

Côté, J. (1999). The influence of the family in the development of talent in sports. *The Sport Psychologist, 13,* 395-417.

Côté, J., Baker, J., & Abernethy, B. (2003). From play to practice: A developmental framework for the acquisition of expertise in team sports. In J. Starkes & K. A. Ericsson (Eds.), *Expert performance in sports: Advances in research on sport expertise* (pp. 89-110). Champaign, IL: Human Kinetics.

Côté, J., Baker, J., & Abernethy, B. (2007). Practice and play in the development of sport expertise. In R. Eklund & G. Tenenbaum (Eds.), *Handbook of sport psychology* (3rd ed., pp. 184-202). Hoboken, NJ: Wiley.

Côté, J., & Fraser-Thomas, J. (2007). Youth involvement in sport. In P. Crocker (Ed.), *Sport psychology: A Canadian perspective* (pp. 270-298). Toronto: Pearson.

Côté, J., & Hay, J. (2002). Children's involvement in sport: A developmental perspective. In J. M. Silva & D. Stevens (Eds.), *Psychological foundations of sport* (2nd ed., pp. 484-502). Boston, MA: Merrill.

Côté, J., MacDonald, D., Baker, J., & Abernethy, B. (2006). When "where" is more important than "when": Birthplace and birthdate effects on the achievement of sporting expertise. *Journal of Sports Sciences, 24,* 217-222.

Ericsson, K. A. (2003). Development of elite performance and deliberate practice: An update from the perspective of the expert performance approach. In J. L. Starkes & K. A. Ericsson (Eds.), *Expert performance in sports: Advances in research on sports expertise* (pp. 49-81). Champaign, IL: Human Kinetics

Ericsson, K. A., Krampe, R. T., & Tesch-Römer, C. (1993). The role of deliberate practice in the acquisition of expert performance. *Psychological Review, 100,* 363-406.

Fraser-Thomas, J., Côté, J., & Deakin, J. (2008a). Examining adolescent sport dropout and prolonged engagement from a developmental perspective. *Journal of Applied Sport Psychology, 20,* 318-333.

Fraser-Thomas, J., Côté, J., & Deakin, J. (2008b). Understanding dropout and prolonged engagement in adolescent competitive sport. *Psychology of Sport and Exercise, 9,* 645-662.

Gould, D. (1987). Understanding attrition in children's sport. In

D. Gould & M. R. Weiss (Eds.), *Advances in pediatric sports sciences* (pp. 61-85). Champaign, IL: Human Kinetics.

Gould, D., & Carson, S. (2004). Fun and games? Myths surrounding the role of youth sports in developing Olympic champions. *Youth Studies Australia, 23,* 19-26.

Gould, D., Feltz, D., Horn, T., & Weiss, M. R. (1982). Reasons for discontinuing involvement in competitive youth swimming. *Journal of Sport Behavior, 5,* 155-165.

Gould, D., & Petlichkoff, L. (1988). Participation motivation and attrition in young athletes. In F. L. Smoll, R. J. Magill, & M. J. Ash (Eds.), *Children in sport* (pp. 161-178). Champaign, IL: Human Kinetics.

Gould, D., Udry, E., Tuffey, S., & Loehr, J. (1996). Burnout in competitive junior tennis players: 1. A quantitative psychological assessment. *The Sport Psychologist, 10,* 322-340.

Hecimovich, M. (2004). Sport specialization in youth: A literature review. *Journal of American Chiropractic Association, 41,* 32-41.

Helsen, W. F., Starkes, J. L., & Hodges, N. J. (1998). Team sports and the theory of deliberate practice. *Journal of Sport & Exercise Psychology, 20,* 12-34.

Hill, G. (1988). Celebrate diversity (not specialization) in school sports. *Executive Educator, 10, 24.*

Hill, G. M., & Hansen, G. F. (1988). Specialization in high school sports—The pros and cons. *Journal of Physical Education, Recreation, & Dance, 59,* 76-79.

Hodge, T., & Deakin, J. (1998). Deliberate practice and expertise in the martial arts: The role of context in motor recall. *Journal of Sport & Exercise Psychology, 20,* 260-279.

Hodges, N. J., & Starkes, J. L. (1996). Wrestling with the nature of expertise: A sport specific test of Ericsson, Krampe and Tesch-Römer's (1993) theory of deliberate practice. *International Journal of Sport Psychology, 27,* 400-424.

King, J., MacDonald, D., Côté, J., & Abernethy, B. (in press). Birthplace effects on the development of female athletic talent. *Journal of Science and Medicine in Sport.*

Kirk, D. (2005). Physical education, youth sport and lifelong participation: The importance of early learning experiences. *European Physical Education Review, 11,* 239-255.

Law, M., Côté, J., & Ericsson, K. A. (2007). Characteristics of expert development in rhythmic gymnastics: A retrospective study. *International Journal of Sport and Exercise Psychology, 5,* 82-103.

Orlick, T., & Botterill, C. (1975). *Every kid can win.* Chicago: Nelson Hall.

Raedeke, T. D. (1997). Is athlete burnout more than just stress? A sport commitment perspective. *Journal of Sport & Exercise Psychology, 19,* 396-417.

Raedeke, T. D., & Smith, A. L. (2001). Development and preliminary validation of an athlete burnout measure. *Journal of Sport & Exercise Psychology, 23,* 281-306.

Régnier, G., Salmela, J., & Russell, S. (1993). Talent detection and development in sport. In N. Singer, M. Murphey, & K. Tennant (Eds.), *Handbook of sport psychology* (1st ed., pp. 290-313). New York: Macmillan.

Robertson-Wilson, J., Baker, J., Derbyshire, E., & Côté, J. (2003). Childhood physical activity involvement in active and inactive female adults. *Avante, 9,* 1-8.

Soberlak, P., & Côté, J. (2003). The developmental activities of elite ice hockey players. *Journal of Applied Sport Psychology, 15,* 41-49.

Starkes, J. L. (2000). The road to expertise: Is practice the only determinant? *International Journal of Sport Psychology, 31,* 431-451.

Starkes, J. L., Deakin, J. M., Allard, F., Hodges, N. J., & Hayes, A. (1996). Deliberate practice in sports: What is it anyway? In K. A. Ericsson (Ed.), *The road to excellence: The acquisition of expert performance in the arts, sciences, sports and games* (pp. 81-106). Mahwah, NJ: Erlbaum.

Wall, M., & Côté, J. (2007). Developmental activities that lead to drop out and investment in sport. *Physical Education and Sport Pedagogy, 12,* 77-87.

Ward, P., Hodges, N. J., Williams, A. M., & Starkes, J. L. (2004). Deliberate practice and expert performance: Defining the path to excellence. In A. M. Williams & N. J. Hodges (Eds.), *Skill acquisition in sport: Research, theory, and practice* (pp. 231-258). New York: Routledge.

Wulf, G., & Shea, C. H. (2002). Principles derived from the study of simple skills do not generalize to complex skill learning. *Psychonomic Bulletin and Review, 9,* 185-222.

Author Note

Support for the writing of this chapter was given by the Social Sciences and Humanities Research Council of Canada (SSHRC Grants # 410-05-1949).

CHAPTER 11

Application of Mental Training with Elite Athletes

RICO SCHUIJERS

In the beginning of the last decade, a compact overview of mental training was provided by Gabler, Janssen, and Nitsch (1990). They discussed the goals, methods, and the subjects involved in mental training. Table 1 gives an overview of mental training based on their work. The first part of this chapter will focus on the work relationship between the sport psychologist and the athlete.

The Sport Psychologist and the Athlete: Procedure

Instructing Mental Skills and the Work Relationship

Mental training is more than the instruction of mental skills. In the literature on applied sport psychology, little information can be found on the work relationship between the sport psychologist (SP) and the athlete (A) (for one example, see Andersen, 2000). To find out more, I turned to psychotherapy and behavioral therapy, where researchers have found that techniques and methods used as psychological interventions have an effect on behavioral changes. However, several other factors also play an important role in the effectiveness of the work relationship. Frank (1974) gave an overview of these factors:

1. The relationship between the SP and the A. The A has confidence in the SP and his or her willingness to help.

2. The office of the SP as a "place of healing." The A feels secure enough there to reveal his or her emotions.

3. Mental training, which helps the A conquer his or her shortcomings.

4. Intervention techniques that are provided by the SP and demonstrate his or her knowledge, and will in turn increase the A's confidence in him or her.

The mental training program always involves a measure of contact between an SP and an A. This can take place individually or in a group. In a group the SP has to teach and instruct in a group setting, with all its advantages (more practical and less time consuming) and disadvantages (less individual attention).

Table 1. An Overview of Mental Training (adapted from Gabler, Janssen, & Nitsch, 1990)

Intention	**Goals**	Increasing action competency	
		Keeping (stabilizing) action competency	
		Minimal deterioration of action competency	
		Recovery of action competency	
		Controlled dismantlement (career ending) of action competency	
	Usefulness	Performance (training in sport)	
		Health (training through sport)	
		Quality of life (self-experience, self-realization, pleasure of life)	
Subject	**Basic accents – individual, and team**	Optimalization of action competency	
		Optimalization of self-influencing and other-influencing action competency	
		Optimalization of movement behavior under conditional, technical, and tactical aspects and/or social behavior (communication and interaction training)	
	Components of action competency	Performance skills	Performance potential
			Stress resistance
			Relaxation skills
			Recovery skills
		Performance readiness	Motivational qualities
			Volitional qualities (willpower)
	Psychological basis of regulation of sports actions	Psychological structures	Internal situation/action representations
			Claims, expectations, prejudices
		Psychological skills for analysis/coping	Optimalization of self-control
			Optimalization of problem solving
Methods	**Methodological point of view**	Etiological and/or symptomatical related processes	
		Motor, psychovegetative, and/or cognitive related processes	
	Intervention way	(Self)-stimulation, -argumentation, -suggestion,- instruction, -knowledge	
		Active doing, observing, visualizing, thinking, (inner) speaking	
	Effectiveness principles	Classic conditioning	
		Operant conditioning	
		Learning through insight	
	Execution form	Individual and/or group training	
		Complete and/or partial training	
		Standardized training and/or adapted training	

Phenomena and events that take place between two people in a "help" setting also apply to a mental training program between an SP and an A. In a Dutch handbook on behavioral therapy (Brinkman, 1978), some general principles and phenomena are discussed. This overview is adapted and adjusted to give an indication of what has to be considered when an SP and an A get together. It is a description of the issues that every SP encounters when he or she is working with elite As.

To complete this picture, a number of psychological models should be mentioned; these can serve as frameworks for the work of SPs. Hill (2001) gives an overview of five models, mentioning the focus and agents of change. The *psychodynamic* model focuses on unconscious inner dynamics and change through insight into personal, unconscious motives. The *behavioral* model focuses on observable behavior and change through learning via conditioning and modeling. The *cognitive* model focuses on thoughts and thought processes and change through how one understands and thinks about the world. The *humanistic* model focuses on subjective experience and change through the support of the

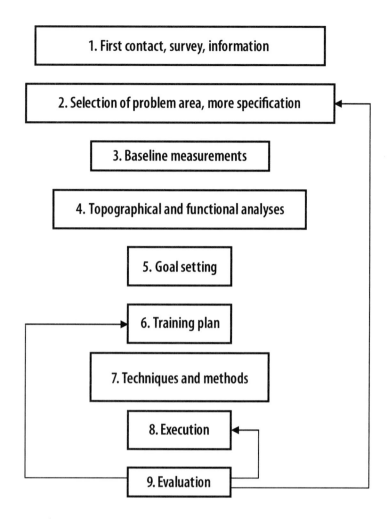

Figure 1. Specific steps in the development of a work relationship between the SP and the A.

individual's natural motivation to seek his or her full potential. The *composite* model Neuro Linguistic Programming (NLP) focuses on how senses are used to create representations of the world and change through the enrichment and alteration of representations. My way of working is cognitive-behavioral based, where other approaches are used if necessary.

The techniques and methods shown in Figure 1, Step 7, are only a small part of the whole process that is needed in the mental training program. In my opinion, the importance of the interaction between the SP and the A has been greatly neglected in sport psychology. One of the few publications on this topic that exist was edited by Andersen (2000). It should be noted that we are not referring to clinical settings but rather normal gatherings of As with SPs.

The First Contact and Basic Conditions

The first contact between an SP and an A usually occurs when the SP is called by the A. The initial questions then arise: Is the request for the caller or for someone else? What is the travelling distance between the two? What is the nature of the complaint? On the basis of these questions, the SP decides either to set up a first meeting or to send him or her to another SP or to another person who can help. If there are no restrictions a day and time can be arranged for the first meeting.

There are two possibilities in the first meeting: common information gathering or, less common, an acute "first aid" meeting. The latter one is chosen when the A is in an acute crisis situation or if the first conversation evokes such heavy emotions that a normal conservation is no longer possible. The common form can vary in structure according to the impression gained by the SP. It can vary from a structured interview to a free association interview in which all the initiative is with the A. Usually a semi-structured interview is chosen, which provides the information the SP wants and at the same time gives room to the A to tell his or her story or to ask questions. There are two main goals: to gather information about the problem of A, and to provide information about the psychological training. A less clear goal is the establishment of a work relationship between the SP and the A. There are several aspects to the first meeting: introduction, beginning of the survey, decision about continuation, giving information about mental training and the roles of the SP and the A, providing the goals and structure of the next session, discussing possible assignments, making agreements, and closing the session.

Regarding the basic conditions of the sessions, three aspects are important: concentration, physical distance, and visibility. Concentration during the sessions can be accomplished easily by making sure there are no disturbances. A red light at the door and unplugging the phone are both ways of assuring that there are no disturbances. An optimal physical distance can be obtained when the A is able to choose between two chairs, each placed at a different distance from the SP. Optimal visibility is ensured when the chairs are low, more or less opposite to each other, and with no desk between them. Gestures of hands and feet are even more visible without any low tables.

The SP and the A shake hands and sit down. The traditional doctor-patient relationship is altered, because a greater degree of intimacy is necessary for effective communication in the mental training. Therefore, it is necessary to determine beforehand how to speak to each other. In English, there is no such thing as a "polite" form of addressing another person—it is always "you." In Dutch you have "u," in German "Sie," and in French "vous." The use of these words creates a distance between two people. To say "je" (in Dutch), "du" (in German), and "tu" (in French) lessens the social distance. The intimacy is intended to help the A feel comfortable enough to reveal personal information, with self-disclosure increasing over time; however, sometimes this has its disadvantages. For example, the A might be threatened by the direct, intimate climate (his or her upbringing taught him or her to be polite). Also, differences in age or social status can make it more difficult for the athlete and psychologist to communicate effectively.

The next step is to gather the necessary basic information, such as name, address, phone number, type of work, etc. It is strongly recommended to tape the first session. The A usually gives a great deal of information and the SP needs his or her energy for listening, thinking, and talking, not for writing down too many things. The SP reveals his or her intention to tape the session ("I always tape my first session, and I intend to do that now"); the motivation for it ("A lot is going to be said, but I can't write it all down; afterwards, I will listen closely to the tape"); informs the A that his or her personal record will be kept confidential ("I listen to the tapes, keep them for a while, and then erase them and use them again"); and asks explicit approval for the taping ("Do you agree to the taping of the first session?"). In almost all cases permission is granted by the A. The A has the fundamental right to refuse, and if this is the case, the conversation will not be recorded.

Beginning of the Survey and Decision about Continuation

Andersen (2000) emphasizes that SPs should help the As to tell their stories. Depending on the educational background of the SP, the conversations can go in different directions. The rational-emotive trained SP will be interested in the As' stories primarily as a source of information about adaptive and maladaptive thinking processes (Ellis, 1994). Client-centered practitioners will listen to personal accounts with an ear for detecting discrepancies between where the As are and where they would like to be (real versus ideal self; Rogers, 1961). Behaviorists (e.g., Wolpe, 1973) will listen to stories for what they say about the As' associations, classical and operant conditioning histories, and current contingencies of reinforcement. Family systems approaches (Hellstedt, 1995) will be concerned with issues such as family homeostasis (the family can also be the team), patterns of communication, hierarchies, and the balance of power. Psychodynamic-oriented SPs (not many of those types are around; see Andersen & Williams-Rice, 1996) will be interested in stories about early experiences, family involvement in the As' sport participation, relationships with coaches and teammates, and how those stories might reveal something about the development of the work relationship between the A and the SP. What you do with the stories you hear, how you interpret them, and where you decide to go with the A in terms of interventions or treatment plans will be determined by the models you choose. The bottom line is helping As tell their stories. Without the stories, you have nothing.

Beginning of the Survey

The SP makes the first move; he or she invites the A to disclose the reason for his or her visit. The answers of the A can vary along two dimensions: the number of problems and the clarity of the formulation. If the A says "When it counts, I fail, I have fear of failure," he or she is mentioning one clear problem. If the A says: "It isn't going as well as it used to," he or she is mentioning one diffuse problem. Other clear problems can be revealed: "My parents put too much pressure on me, my teammates ignore me, and my coach doesn't give me confidence," or more diffuse problems: "Everything is going wrong, I am getting old, I can't handle it anymore." The SP can ask for more clarity in the case of diffuse problems. The five questions that should be raised for every problem are listed and described in Table 2.

In this stage the conversation techniques are mainly the use of open questions, and "going along with the A." One extensive answer to an open question often reveals more information than a dozen questions to which the answer is "yes" or "no." The kind of answers the A gives to an open question suggests to what extent the A has thought about his or her problem and how well he or she can keep track of it. Sometimes the problem "floats" over to another problem during the answering of the first question. "Well, I told you about the tension during the games where my father was watching, but actually I am always tense when my father is around, I wonder what he thinks of me, if he loves me…" Often, these diversions occurring in the A's thoughts will reveal underlying causalities of the problem. "The tension in the games started when my girlfriend complained about my absence because of my sport activities. She said she was going to do more things by herself. I worry now that I don't give her much attention, and maybe she will start seeing a lover. I can't bear the idea of a lover, and it makes me tense in games." Another kind of "flotation" in the answers can be toward total irrelevance. For example, "I moved from the south to the north, and started to play there. From the first moment I felt enormous tension, also because of the mentality of the people. I don't know if you know, but those people are so different, for example, I walked through town and…" These kinds of answers do not give clear information about the problem, but they do give information about the A. When the initial response is given, the SP has techniques to keep the A focused on providing relevant information about the problem or to get the A back on track when he or she has floated away during the first answer. These techniques include repetitions, positive reinforcement, abstracts, and interpretations.

Repetitions, the repeating of what the A says by paraphrasing and reflecting, serve both as a signal that the SP is still listening and accepting, and as encouragement to go on. *Positive reinforcement* can be given verbally by words like "yes," and "I understand." It can also be given by nodding yes with the head as a non-verbal

Table 2. Questions for Clarification of the Problem

What is the content of the problem?	The SP tries together with the A to make the problem understood by both of them. This means that the SP tries to learn the "language" the A uses (what does he or she mean by "failure," when does he or she experience pressure, etc.)
Since when?	To get a global idea of how long the A has had the complaint, the SP should ask for a short history.
What are the causes or facilitators?	Sometimes the A gives clear causes for his or her problem. "After missing that penalty shot, I have felt tension at important moments." In other cases the causes and facilitators are not as clear: "I don't know why this has become more severe lately."
What is the seriousness of the problem?	What are the consequences for the A, the family, the club, or the country (in case of a national team player)? The SP tries to get a picture of the consequences of the complaint as well as the reactions to those consequences by the A and significant others.
When does problem behavior occur?	Can it be predicted when the behavior will take place?

positive reinforcement. The SP uses his or her communication skills to repeat or reinforce relevant information given by the A.

Abstracts made by the SP establish the essence of the A's statements. These summaries make it possible to change the subject in the session if necessary or appropriate or to to check if the SP understood the A correctly. If not the topic can be clarified. *Interpretations* can make a long story short and clear. They provide an overview of what the A has said. Interpretations can vary in three ways: depth, clarity, and positiveness (sureness). Interpretations are hypotheses formed by the SP regarding events and/or causal relationships of events in the present or recent past of the A. The clearer the hypotheses, the better the A can discuss the matter.

In addition to the information that is given through questions and answers, there are other aspects of the interaction that strongly influence its progress. These include all the non-verbal elements, such as gestures and characteristics of speech. Three elements will be discussed here: the attention of the SP, his or her friendliness, and the amount of tension.

The *attention* of the SP can be demonstrated through concrete gestures, of which the most important are frequency of nodding "yes," turning the head and body toward the A, frequency of eye contact, and the frequency of movements of the fingers and hands and the legs and feet. By showing optimal attention, the SP appears friendly, which creates a positive rapport that helps to reveal the A's degree of comfort with self-disclosure and facilitates the A's willingness to proceed in conversation.

The perceived *friendliness* of the SP by the A is determined by the SP's nodding and turning toward the A, but also in the smile-frequency and the number of positive remarks. However, it is important not to overdo this behavior, because the SP has to stay authentic. Usually there isn't much to smile about, because the A tells about problems and complaints he or she has. It is erroneous for the SP to feel that he or she should be friendly at all times and always radiate warmth; sometimes he or she has to be more strict.

The amount of *tension* can be indicated by frequency of object manipulation (playing with a pen; plucking a hair, moustache, or beard; tapping fingers); tense positions (legs stiffly closed, heels lifted off the floor, hands placed in armpits, shoulders put forward, sitting on the edge of the seat); and a slow talking pace and long periods of silence. Tension and fear felt by the SP evokes tension and fear in the A. Some characteristics of speech are very important: (a) the speed (not too slow, not too fast); (b) volume; (c) modulation (not speaking in one tone); (d) clear "punctuation" (a question is a spoken as a question, sentences have definite endings); (e) absence of irrelevant noises or stress on parts of words, no "uh's" or throat noises; (f) absence of interruptions (taking care not to speak until the A has finished his or her sentence); (g) maximal clarity of language (no difficult words, no long sentences); (h) no long, uncomfortable silences.

An optimal style of the SP, using the charateristics mentioned above, both in verbal and in non-verbal behavior, not only makes the first contact easier, but also provides the A with an adequate model for social interaction—verbally and non-verbally. By being calm and relaxed, clear, non-aggressive, and non-evaluative, the SP can provide an important example of positive interaction.

Decision about Continuation

After the first survey, a decision has to be made about the continuation of the training. The list presented here is not complete, but gives an idea why some A's do not continue (see Table 3).

Providing Information on Mental Training and the Roles of the SP and the A

The SP and the A comprise a small, task-directed, functioning group. This group functions better if the goals are known and accepted and the way of working is clear. In the first place, the A should have an understanding of mental training: It is concrete, and aimed at the present problems or skills. The objective of mental training is to know, understand, and solve the problems of the A. The A is a co-worker of the SP, and decisions are made together. Second, the SP makes the structure of the mental training clear without going into too much detail. The first step in explaining the structure of the mental training is that the survey of the complaints is made, and then a problem is chosen. Then, this problem is worked on further. The second step is that the SP makes a training plan, which is continuously adjusted on the basis of the results. The third step is that the SP describes his or her role, the A's role, and what is expected of the A: to be on time, talk clearly, work hard during the sessions, do the homework, protest, criticize, and ask questions when necessary according to the A's

Table 3. Possible Reasons for Not Continuing the Mental Training Program

The problem is not psychological in nature
The problem is determined by organic reasons, for example, an injury
The complaints are severe but normal according to the situation, for example, a slump in the performance because of the death of a family member
The problem is too serious for a SP
The problem is too serious for this SP, with countertransference, for example
The A prefers another kind of training
The A cannot afford the cost of the training

perceptions. The A can point out if friction occurs, so that there can be a possibility of discussing it.

Closing the First Meeting. In the final minutes of the first session homework can be given, the goals and structure of the next sessions are provided, agreements are made. The SP provides the structure of the mental training, including factors such as fees, length of time, regularity, homework, and ethics, and then closes the first session. In addition, questionnaires can be given. The questionnaires include personality tests and tests for psychological characteristics such as fear of failure and coping with problems. The results of these tests are interpreted and written down in a sport psychological profile. The information of this profile is used in the mental training by focusing more on some skills because that is better for this A.

Processing the Material from the First Meeting

Questionnaires offer the SP valuable official information about the A, from which he or she can build hypotheses and ideas about a particular A. There is also a large amount of unofficial information received by the SP, such as the non-verbal behavior of the A. Sometimes non-verbal actions and verbal statements are compatible, and sometimes they contradict. For example, when an A says he is happy but his body language is that his face is not happy and he is looking down to the ground. Furthermore, the SP also receives signals from his or her own body: it becomes warm, he or she doesn't feel comfortable, or feels scared or sad, when the A is aggressive or when the story of the A is full of misery and bad luck. Emotional reactions can be provoked by thoughts such as "she annoys me" or "I don't like him." Memories of

other As spontaneously can occur. The information collected from the A, along with the SP's signals, is important, although it can cause disruptions in the training, and can interfere with the original goal of the training. Such information is often neglected as not scientifically useful; however, this is a mistake. This information can be very important and useful for the effectiveness of the communication between the SP and the A, although there is no model for it. The following are some recommendations for dealing with this information: (a) formulate the most obvious information abstractly; (b) detect the differences between official and non-official information; (c) determine possible links between the information and the problems of the A; (d) try to put important observations into a direct question; and (e) determine if these observations have implications for the behavior of the SP in the following sessions.

In this regard, transference and countertransference from the psychodynamic approach should be mentioned concerning the relationship between the SP and the A. *Transference* is when As begin to respond to SPs either in ways similar to how they have responded to significant others in the past (e.g., parents) or in ways they would like to respond to fantasized figures (e.g., the good father they never had). *Countertransference* is when similar transferring of past responses, perceptions, and behaviors occurs on the part of the SP and is directed toward the A. Both transference and countertransference give information that is important for the mental training, in either a negative or positive manner.

Topographical Analysis. Based on the information from the conversations, a topographical analysis can be made. In this analysis the SP tries to obtain an accurate image of the problematic behavior and the situation(s) in which it occurs. The SP can ask direct questions to make the problem more clear ("This choking, can you tell me more about it?"), or can merely observe the A. In this analysis the main goal is to get the problem of the A to become more clear.

Some problems can occur in the topographical analysis, such as when emotions, moods, thoughts, and other private events are revealed. This is not useful in this stage because the topographical analysis has only to do with behavior. Sometimes an A has to express the emotional and cognitive processes that are going on in order to grasp the importance of the stimuli that are causing the problem behavior. Another obstacle can occur when the A is not providing useful or relevant information. This can be caused by several factors. One, the SP might exhibit poor conversation technique; if he or she is unable to ask the right questions, there will be a lack of information or a failure to compel the A to think further. Two, the A might withhold vital information; typically, this is not a deliberate act, but might be a result of shame or guilt felt by the A. Three, the A has nothing left to tell. When there is nothing more to tell the SP, the SP must continue with the next part of the session.

Finally, a problem can arise when the SP does not keep in mind the essence of the topograpical analysis. That is, he or she is too quick with behaviors like advising, comforting, finding solutions, and giving short-term tips. These behaviors are not well thought through, and can be very dysfunctional for the process of the mental training. In the beginnning the topographical analysis can be unclear or incomplete. However, during subsequent sessions some vital information can come forward.

Functional Analysis. The functional analysis can be made based on the same material derived from the questions and observations as that used in the topographical analysis. In this analysis, the SP connects the complaints and problems with the consequences and the predictors or facilitators. There are three ways in which the problem behavior can occur:

(1) The problem behavior can be a conditioned response to a stimulus, which the SP tries to discover. For example, seeing an opponent on the pitch evokes feelings of anxiety and causes attempts to flee.

(2) The problem behavior can be operant behavior; the SP and the A look then for discriminative stimuli. This means looking for influential factors. For example, a boy who normally is agitated and enthusiastic during the game becomes aggressive and negative when his parents are watching.

(3) The problem behavior can be positively and negatively reinforced. The problem behavior can be swearing, hitting, or annoying other players during practice and in competition. A reward can be the attention of the coach, even if it is in a negative way. If this problem behavior is rewarded, it will last longer.

An adequate functional analysis is empirical (similar to the events in everyday life), complex (many factors determining the problem behavior), and individualized (general qualities of people are compared with those of one person). The function of this analysis is for the SP to switch from information-gathering to setting goals and designing a training plan. For the A, the functional analysis has two functions: (1) it facilitates greater insight into the problem ; and (2) it encourages the A to model the cognitive style and way of thinking of the SP.

Based on both the topographical and the functional analyses, the SP can begin to build a theory about the problem behavior of the A, which will include a discussion of the problem, the specific stimuli that cause certain behaviors and responses, and why this occurs.

Goal Setting, Training Plan, and Evaluation
Goal Setting. Not only is goal setting a technique used in mental training for handling the problems of the A, but it is a necessary part of the structure of the mental training itself. First, goals should be set that consider the outcome (dependent) variables, such as the execution of movements in an effective way, or the performance. Second, goals should be set for the mental skills (independent variables). These goals should be set such that they can be measured and scored.

When many goals have to be set, it is impossible to work on them simultaneously. Therefore, choices must be made. Some guidelines and considerations for choosing the appropriate goal: (a) the certainty of the relationship between the dependent and independent variables must be established; (b) some relations between dependent and independent variables are more important than others; (c) some goals can be of more general use than others; (d) some goals should be accomplished first so that the next problem can be taken on; and (e) some goals are easier to reach than others. Based on these guidelines, the SP and A can choose the most productive and efficient time to work on each goal.

In goal setting, three major difficulties can occur: (a) the problem seems to be unsolvable, because all the goals for the independent variables are not reachable; (b) the people involved in the training (for example, in a team) do not agree on the goals that are being set; and (c) the A finds all the goals irrelevant to the current problem. In these cases, the SP tries to find solutions that are acceptable to the A. He or she does not force the A to accept his or her own ideas of the goal setting, but instead talks, analyzes, and tries to give a model to the A for problem-solving behavior.

Training Plan. Based on the goals for the independent variables, a training plan can be made. Planning consists of two parts: (a) determining for each goal if it concerns learning or unlearning and if it requires respondent, overt, or covert behavior; and (b) choosing which techniques and methods can work for the learning or unlearning of the respondent, overt, or covert behavior.

In this way, a 3 x 2 classification schema can be made (see Table 4). Learning can be divided into acquisition of

new behavior and increasing the frequency of new behavior. Acquisition, increasing frequency, and unlearning are three dimensions of the learning/unlearning side of changing behavior. The two on the other end include overt/covert behavior and respondent behavior. For each combination there is a technique or method that is most effective.

The list of the techniques and methods presented in Table 4 is not complete, and some techniques are on the same dimension, or can be used for another kind of goal. The choice of the techniques depends on a few variables. The first is, of course, the nature of the problem, and then learning or unlearning of overt, covert, or respondent behavior. The choice can be made on several grounds:

(1) The literature shows that technique x has a better chance for success in population y, and if the A belongs to population y, then technique x is preferable.

(2) When there is no other way to predict success, the SP chooses a technique based on his or her experience.

(3) When the SP is more comfortable with technique x than technique y, technique x should be used.

Table 4. Classification Schema for Changing Behavior

		Overt/Covert behavior	Respondant behavior
Learning	Acquisition of new behavior	Operant conditioning Shaping Modeling Stimulus discrimination	Classic conditioning Emotional training B
	Increasing frequency of behavior	Contingency management Prompting Stimulus discrimination C	Removing inhibitions Stimulus control D
Unlearning	Reducing frequency of behavior	Extinction Punishment Negative practice Thought stopping E	Flooding Counter-conditioning Systematic desensitization F

(4) When no theoretical background or valid data can be found about a technique, then this technique should not be used.

(5) It is preferable to use techniques that are less time-consuming.

(6) Techniques that are less painful or annoying to the A are preferable.

In choosing the right techniques or methods, the SP should be aware that he or she should not use only quick techniques, such as thought stopping and relaxation training. In doing so, the SP would give the impression that a problem can be quickly solved by relaxing and not thinking about it, which sometimes is not in harmony with reality. In applying techniques and methods, the SP should be realistic at all times.

Evaluation. In the evaluation session, usually three questions are asked: (a) What has changed in the complaint we worked on during the last sessions, and why?; (b) What have you learned from this mental training program so far?; and (c) Are there changes in other problems that we did discuss, or have new problems arisen?

What has changed in the complaint we worked on during the last sessions and why? Usually the answers of the A are consistent with the conclusions of the SP, but sometimes the A is less positive than the SP would have expected. Occasionally the termination of a problem evokes the feeling of *loss*, and therefore can cause depressed feelings. This is especially so when the complaint had a function in the advantage the A had in using this complaint to avoid situations and maintain self-esteem. Answers to the second part of the question (i.e., why?) differ greatly. Some refer to the SP, some to the processes between the SP and the A, and some to the content of the mental training program.

What have you learned from this mental training program so far? As can mention the separate skills or achieved insights about their behavior, and their causes. Some answers have nothing to do with the content of the mental training program, but they are opinions about some basic facts of life that are mentioned by the A. For example, "My athletic career is shot," and "Why do I worry so much?"

Are there changes in other, not directly discussed problems, or have new problems arisen? Depending on the answers to other questions that can be asked, such as, "Will we still work on this problem, or choose another?" or "Can we end the mental training?" the SP will tell the A what is indicated if the mental training program continues with another objective.

Processes between the Sport Psychologist and the Athlete

The process between the SP and the A can be divided into (1) the development of the work relationship, and (2) the work problems that can occur in the mental training.

Development of the Work Relationship between the SP and the A

In the beginning, the SP tries to build up a good work relationship with the A. The SP wants to build a "team" with the A in order to strive for a goal (reducing or eliminating the problems of the A) in a direct way. Initially there are no intense mutual feelings of appreciation or conflict. The work relationship changes over time, and is influenced by three processes: self-disclosure, emotion-inducing stimuli, and other aspirations for the work relationship.

Much self-disclosure by the A confers an increase in intimacy, because the information that the A gives to the SP can be highly personal. Often this information has not been revealed previously to anyone. This is the kind of information that is normally shared with intimate others. The SP can become in a way one of these intimate others—not all the way, though. Two important features of an intimate relationship are lacking in an SP-A relationship. First, no other intimate behavior takes place between the two. No dinners together, no caressing, no kissing, no sleeping with each other. Second, the relationship is very unequal. The A tells the SP many intimate things, but the SP divulges very little about himself or herself to the A.

The SP and A are constantly giving *emotion-inducing stimuli* to one another. The SP constantly gives positive reinforcement; he or she listens, is understanding, and is rewarding. An SP who reinforces often, gives attention, and is accepting becomes himself or herself a positive conditioned stimulus. But the SP is also a person, a stimulus, who is a reinforcer of negative feelings and experiences. The SP is always a reinforcer of both positive as well as negative feelings. It must be realized that the SP provides a great deal of stimuli to the A that are emotionally-loaded. In addition, the A can praise the SP by telling him or her that he or she is the best and that the method the SP is using works the best. The A can also relate negative feelings to the SP, by saying, for example, that he or she is uncertain if the training will ever work. In addition, the SP has his or her own history, which induces the emotions that are evoked from the remarks of the A. The SP who is uncertain about himself or herself can have negative emotions such as aggression, anxiety, and grief after a negative remark from the A. The SP might think back to earlier experiences; that is, he or she brings his or her past to the sessions. However, it would be better if the SP recognizes this and copes with these feelings in order to remain focused on this particular A.

SP and A often have *other wishes* for the work relationship. There is an agreement between the SP and A which is as follows: "We started this training to work on your problems as an athlete." The official wish of the A is, "I want to get rid of my problems," and of the SP is, "I want help you to get rid of your problems." But the SP and the A are people who also have social interests; for example, to be liked or loved, to be passive, to be angry and aggressive, to be full of revenge, or to beat everyone else. The SP can also have wishes in daily life that influence the relationship with the A.

The wishes (coming from deprivations and needs) can differ in intensity, consciousness (the clearness of the wish), acceptability, and generality or specificity. Deprivations determine needs, needs determine wishes, and wishes determine search behavior. Within a need all search behavior is functionally identical; they have the same stimuli and the same reinforcers. For example, deprivation of food leads people to search behavior that is activated by the same stimulus (feeling hungry) and is reinforced by functional identical stimuli (eatable goods), but the situation will determine the kind of search behavior that is exhibited. Feeling hungry in a forest will evoke behavior different than feeling hungry in a city. Characteristics of the wish itself are also important for the kind of behavior that is shown. With a high intensity wish, the behavior is quick, long lasting, and intense. With specific wishes, the search behavior differs from that for general wishes. With conscious wishes, the search behavior is structured and directed, otherwise it is diffuse.

The A brings along wishes he or she has in life. For example, he or she can have the intense wish to be liked by everybody, and will take this wish to the training. To gain the sympathy of the SP, the A can praise the SP, work hard, or make the SP feel pity by telling the sadness of the situation over and over again. These are different forms of search behavior for the same wish (to be liked by the SP). Some of these behaviors are compatible with adequate training behavior, others are not. Praising and complaining are not compatible with adequate training behavior. Working hard is compatible. If it is compatible the SP will reinforce that behavior, which will increase the positive attitude toward the SP. If the search behavior is not compatible with the training behavior, the SP will discourage or punish this behavior. This can lead to frustration and a negative attitude toward the SP.

Search behavior for the unofficial wishes of the A can appear in different forms, as can the emotions that are induced by the SP's behavior. Globally, the wishes can appear in three forms:

(1) *Relational wishes* and problems can appear as work problems (see next paragraph). Not committing to the homework, calling to cancel five minutes before the start of a session, or arriving late for a session can be behavior by an A with a wish to make the SP angry. An A with a wish to be passive-aggressive can give a lot of "don't know" answers, does not want to fully commit to the skills or homework, and asks if the homework assignments can be changed.

(2) *Irrelevant questions* are comprised of very overt and short, not work-relevant questions, remarks, and nonverbal behaviors. A lonely A asks, "You never go for dinner with your As, do you?" when she has a desire for an affectionate relationship. Other irrelevant questions and remarks are, for example, that an A with a tic in the face can show this tic more overtly after the announcement that the SP is going on a holiday. The A feels deserted and reveals this by showing the tic. This is irrelevant for the effectiveness of the training process. Other behavior is giving presents. The kind of presents often reveals the motive for giving a present, for example, giving the SP the favorite music of the A. It is best to stop these behaviors by not giving much notice to them.

(3) *Reports about consequences of the sessions,* that is, what happened after the previous session, for example a headache after the session. For an A, a headache after a session in which he or she talked about stressful things can be seen as a sign of relieving tension, but is an unpleasant feeling. The SP knows that it is good for the A to let go of the tension through a headache, but is also punished because the A tells him or her that the only thing she gets from the training is a headache.

Mistakes and Work Problems in the Mental Training and Coping with Work Problems

Mistakes can be made by the SP in the first contact. Usually this is caused by an irrational desire to help and the opinion that mental training should be short and effective. Some other mistakes are caused by inexperience. For example, *giving unsolicited advice* is ineffective at all times. In this situation the mental training does not exceed the level of casual social conversation, as in a bar or other public gathering place, and does not often provide help for the A's problem. The giving of advice that doesn't address the seriousness of the complaint and the uniqueness of the A is not beneficial. The same goes for *talking away,* or an unwanted relativization of the problem: "Everybody has fear sometimes," and "Most people are a little bit crazy." This can belittle the A, can evoke aggression, and is detrimental to the building of a good work relationship. A third mistake is to make *unasked optimistic predictions,* such as "Within no time you will be free of this fear of failure," or "I can give you more self-confidence." The SP does not know enough from one session to make predictions like this, and at the same time he or she is building up expectations. Another mistake is to apply *therapeutic actions* too quickly, like giving relaxation training in the first session.

Many mistakes are made because some SPs don't perceive surveying, listening, or clarification as essential elements of training. The opposite is true. The A comes for mental training because he or she did not succeed in coping with his or her problems for a long period of time, often because he or she could not make the first steps, survey, or formulate an overview of the problem(s). By discussing the problems, the training has already started.

In addition, SPs might commit the error of *making value judgments* and *not answering As' questions adequately.* Making value judgments plays a role in the mental training, but should be avoided in the first meeting because it can evoke aggression and a feeling of not being understood. The questions of the A can involve technical matters ("How does the relaxation training work?"), can involve the SP ("How old are you?"), or be about the A ("Can my problem be treated anyway?"). Questions vary along two dimensions: the *intimacy value* and the *answerability.* Questions of the A should be answered in a short and clear manner. It is undesirable to be evasive ("We'll come back to that later"), to avoid counter-questions ("Why are you asking me that now?"), to insert interpretations ("Asking these questions comes from your insecurity"), or to directly or indirectly refuse to respond ("That is none of your business"). When the SP doesn't know the answer to a question the A asks, he or she should merely reply "I don't know." Clear answers are a model for the question-answer behavior that the SP expects from the A, and this reduces the feeling of a doctor-patient relationship. The hardest questions to answer for the SP are questions that are highly intimate, usually about impressions of the SP of the A. ("People say I am very shy and quiet, you have seen me now for an hour, do you feel the same about me?"). An "I don't know" answer is unlikely because the SP is supposed to be an expert on these kinds of matters. The SP can best answer this question by giving his or her impression of the A, adding the fact that he or she is seeking help for this problem, that the SP has a fundamental approach of accepting people regardless of what they reveal, and that accepting and taking people as they are is a part of an SP's work. Questions asked by the As are by definition not irrelevant. They serve the purpose of reducing uncertainties, testing the credibility of the SP, and finding ways to get closer to the SP and the problem without fear.

Problems During the Mental Training

Difficulties occur when the A behaves in a way that is incompatible with behaviors that lead to an effective conversation. The A then evokes disturbing emotional reactions from the SP. No proper conversation can be started with an A who comes in, moves the chair to a corner, and is silent. Other behavior is less obvious but still disturbing, such as continuous and irrelevant talking, intense emotional reactions (incessant crying), and extremely dominant behavior (taking over the lead). Such behaviors evoke emotional responses in the SP. He or she can become frightened because of the intensity of the emotions, or can feel insecure when his or her schedule for the first meeting is so bluntly disturbed, and is annoyed by these disturbances.

The best way to handle these situations is to lower the emotional responses through mental relaxation techniques (those that the A still must learn) and leave behind every form of social punishment (the experiences of the A are probably caused by punishment that has not been effective). The SP has some alternative reactions. First, he or she can passively allow the emotions of the A to dissipate, thus using social extinction. Second, in the short breaks for breathing, the SP can ask brief questions that require a short answer, giving some direction to the conversation. Third, the SP can use powerful confrontation methods by naming the unwanted behavior ("You are answering in a long way"), expressing his or her wish ("Could you answer more briefly?"), or inviting the A to do something ("Could you do that for me?").

Coping with Work Problems

It is not entirely clear how the behaviors and emotions of the A can enhance or decrease the efficiency of the training process. This is dependent on how and what the SP does when they intervene. There are four ways to cope with relational problems between the SP and the A and the emotions that go along with them. In the first, the SP analyzes the difficulties, and changes his or her behavior toward the A. The second way is to discuss the work problems. The third way is talking about remarks and behaviors that are not task-relevant. The fourth way is having an explicit, substantial discussion about what is happening between the SP and the A during an evaluation session.

(1) *The SP changes his or her behavior.* It is advisable to always start with this approach. The SP can become aware of the negative emotions he or she is experiencing toward the A, make a mini-functional analysis of where the feelings come from, and determine which stimuli evoke these emotions. He or she can formulate methods to prevent these stimuli from occuring by changing his or her own behavior during the session. With difficult As, this process will occur often. Sometimes modifications in behavior will not lead to the desired changes, so that this hypothesis could be wrong. This

way of coping with the relational problems assumes that the SP is also a factor in these troubles, that he or she also has shortcomings, and that it is unjust to blame all the troubles on the A.

(2) *Solve relational problems.* Relational problems can manifest themselves in work problems. A work problem is defined as behavior that is related to the sessions themselves. For example, after feeling angry in a session, an A goes directly to a candy store to buy sweets. This behavior can be discussed in one of the subsequent sessions. The discussion of what happened can provide insight into the A's behavior. The A should differentiate between training sessions and everyday life. After a while he or she can generalize the behavior from the training session to the outside world. The purpose is not to gain insight per se, but to produce insight through one's own volition. New, learned behavior can often counteract old, existing behavior.

(3) *Avoid relationships outside the work relationship.* Wishes and emotions can be revealed to the SP by verbal and non-verbal behavior outside the work relationship. SPs and As also see each other outside the office of the SP, for example, on the venue. The A can sometimes show inappropriate behavior outside the hour of the session. The SP should be aware of what the A is trying to do and stop it right away. Signals are clearer when the distance between what is said or done and what is "actually" meant is minimal. The distance between "You never have dinner with an A, do you?" and "You don't want to have dinner with me, I suppose?" is smaller and the SP can bring this question into discussion. The first aim, then, is to find out what the A is "really" saying, by means of asking questions. It is advisable to handle these kinds of remarks with care and not to allow the interpretation of the SP to be shown too directly. Often a direct question, such as "Do you want to have dinner with me?" is

too threatening. On the other hand, there is a strong desire to ask the question. This approaching-avoiding conflict results in the statement of compromise: "You never have dinner with As, do you?" A direct question can lead to direct avoidance and denial behavior. The answers of the A can be immediate. In that case it is wiser to let it rest. Questions and remarks that have nothing to do with training or that are already clear to the SP should be directly answered at the same level.

(4) *Solve problems during evaluation sessions.* Finally, problems between SP and A can occur during the evaluation sessions. "How are we doing so far?" is the question that is asked here. An A can give an answer on the work level, such as, "I want to talk more instead of doing exercises." The SP can relate to this and tell the A that they will spend more time doing the things he or she wants. If the A expresses a clear relational problem with the SP, which is not put forth quickly or is not sufficiently discussed, this is a serious matter. The problem should be made specific, the background explored, and an attempt made to find solutions. Suppose the A tells the SP hesitantly that he or she has the feeling that the SP "does not like me." Making the problem specific is accomplished by asking questions such as "Since when do you feel that way?" and "What are the things I do that make you feel that way?" The opinions of As are seldom totally inaccurate; usually, some of the things the A says are true—perhaps not as extreme as the A thinks, but they do exist. For example, the SP can notice that indeed the A does not appreciate his or her efforts anymore. He or she has the feeling that the A does not want the training and the A's behavior is counterproductive, which is irritating to the SP. It is important for the SP to relate these findings to the A, even if they are very painful, and to determine, together with the A, if these perceptions are true. Only when both have the same

image of the problems it is appropriate to search for solutions. These agreements should consider both the A and the SP, because the determinants for relational problems lie with both of them. Sometimes the A reports a feeling during evaluation that existed previously, but is no longer relevant. This can be treated in the same way as the remarks discussed earlier.

Final Remarks about the Relationship Between the SP and the A

The relationship between an SP and an A often changes from a neutral work relationship to a more complex one. The goal of the SP is to establish an optimal work relationship with the A. This work relation is aimed at specific training goals: diminishing or eliminating complaints and the learning of skills by the A so that he or she can cope with future obstacles more independently. The relationship is formalized on strictly set times and days. Furthermore, there is no other contact between the SP and the A. They do not visit each other, or go to a movie together; they do not drink, eat, or sleep with each other. When the SP-A relationship is closest to an optimal work relationship, the training will develop positively, and the affinity between the SP and the A will be productive. It is clear what can and cannot be done in a mental training relationship. The SP tries, without relenting, to be a model for adequate behavior in such a work relationship. This means occluding his or her own emotions unless they are task-relevant. Feelings of anger or of being in love, for example, should not be brought into the work relationship between the SP and the A. These feelings should indeed be recognized and worked on by the SP (either by himself or herself, in supervision, or in his or her own training). If these feelings cannot be coped with in an acceptable way, they will greatly disturb the work relationship. In those cases it is advisable to cancel the mental training after an explanation of why this decision was made.

It is very important to note that all of the elements mentioned in this chapter about the relationship between the SP and the A, from the moment of the first telephone call to the end of the training, are valid for all SPs. These processes and decisions are experienced by every SP; however, relationships between SPs and As can be differentiated by the amount or the intensity of the experienced processes.

References

Andersen, M. B. (2000). Beginnings: Intakes and the initiation of relationships. In M. B. Andersen (Ed.), *Doing sport psychology* (pp. 3-16). Champaign, IL: Human Kinetics.

Andersen, M. B., & Williams-Rice, B. T. (1996). Supervision in the education and training of sport psychology service providers. *The Sport Psychologist, 10,* 278-290.

Brinkman, W. (1978). Het gedragtherapeutisch proces [The behavioral therapeutic process]. In J. W. G. Orlemans (Ed.), *Handboek gedragstherapie* [Handbook of behavioral therapy] (pp. 1-60). Losbladige editie [edition] 1978-1992. Deventer: Van Loghum Slaterus.

Ellis, A. (1994). The sport of avoiding sports and exercise: A rational-emotive behavior therapy perspective. *The Sport Psychologist, 8,* 248-261.

Frank, J. D. (1974). *Persuasion and healing: A comparative study of psychotherapy* (Rev. ed.). New York: Schocken Books.

Gabler, H., Janssen, J.-P., & Nitsch, J. R. (1990). *Gutachten "Psychologisches Training" in der Praxis des Leistungssports. Probleme und Perspektiven.* Köln: Sport und Buch Strauss.

Hellstedt, J. C. (1995). Invisible players: A family systems model. In S. M. Murphy (Ed.), *Sport psychology interventions* (pp. 117-147). Champaign, IL: Human Kinetics.

Hill, K. L. (2001). *Frameworks for sport psychologists.* Champaign, IL: Human Kinetics.

Rogers, C. R. (1961). *On becoming a person.* Boston: Houghton Mifflin.

Wolpe, J. (1973). *The practice of behavior therapy* (2nd ed.). New York: Pergamon.

CHAPTER 12

Regulating Mental States through Electroencephalography and Heart Rate Biofeedback Training

TSUNG-MIN HUNG, DONG-YANG FONG, YUNG-SHUN WANG, PO-YI LIN, AND LI-CHUAN LO

In the few seconds prior to motor skill execution, an athlete's mental state is critical to performance in areas such as attention and arousal (Salazar et al., 1990). This is especially true in sports and sport activities such as archery, rifle shooting, golf putting, and basketball free throws. The athlete's attention is particularly vulnerable to internal interference by task-irrelevant thought due to the self-paced nature of these activities (Boutcher, 1992). The interference is even more significant when athletes are under stress. Robazza, Bortoli, and Nougier (2000) observed in a case study that the archer never abandoned a shot in practice; however, the archer abandoned an average of 1.5 out of every 6 shots in competition. The archer also performed much more poorly in competition than in practice. This clearly illustrates that competition stress has a toll on an athlete's mental state, resulting in underperformance.

Understanding of optimal mental states is the first step in helping athletes control their mind during sport performance. Research has suggested that peak performance can be characterized by indicators such as lack of negative self-talk (Meichenbaum, 1977), high self-efficacy (Feltz, 1984), adapting and attention to task-relevant cues when facing challenges (Landers, 1980), and a feeling of flow. The athlete's skill in competition is usually developed through numerous training sessions, and is a result of adaptation to the challenge imposed by the environment. Thus, it is necessary to examine optimal mental states with consideration given to how the athlete physically and mentally adapts to his or her environment. Hatfield and Hillman (2001) suggest that optimal mental states increase the probability of performance efficiency and can reach the state of automaticity proposed by Fitts and Posner (1967). These states also help the performer filter out interference from task irrelevant cognitive and emotional processes.

Seeking ways to assist athletes to reach their peak is a long-term effort for sport psychologists. Psychological skills such as arousal regulation, goal setting, self-confidence, concentration, and self-talk seem to be effective in performance enhancement (Weinberg & Gould, 2007). The content of psychological skill training (PST) varies for individual athletes, various sports, and level of skills. Biofeedback training, one of the techniques in PST, has been applied mostly for arousal regulation and relaxation. However, biofeedback is also effective for enhancing concentration and reducing the effects of interference. This in turn can enhance the sense of control over one's mental state. The purposes of this chapter are to (1) briefly introduce biofeedback, and (2) review studies utilizing neurofeedback training and heart rate (HR) biofeedback training to enhance sport performance.

Biofeedback

Theoretical Background

The concept of biofeedback originated in late 1960. Biofeedback is now applied in many fields, such as rehabilitation, educational correction, psychotherapy, and athletic training (Moss, 1994). Researchers view biofeedback from different perspectives. Some focus on the involvement of the process, while others consider the importance of the goals of biofeedback. Still, there are researchers who maintain the importance of combining elements from both the methodology and the purposes of biofeedback. The process-focused researchers define biofeedback as an experiment of applying an external sensor to provide real time bodily process of an organism (Schwartz & Beatty, 1977). The purpose-focused researchers believe that the goal of biofeedback is to enhance the self-control capacity of an individual within his or her physiological processes (Ray, Raczynski, Rogers, & Kimball, 1979). The combination-focused researchers consider biofeedback to be a way of analyzing the physiological condition of an individual with certain equipment and helping the individual learn how to manipulate the physiological information by visual or auditory signal (Basmajian, 1978).

There are three steps involved in biofeedback training (Blanchard & Goodstein, 1978). The first is the detection and amplification of bio-signals. Bio-signals, such as electroencephalography (EEG), electromyography (EMG), and HR, are so small that untrained individuals are usually unaware of any changes they undergo. However, the electronic device can easily detect the minor changes and amplify them for analysis.

The second step is to transform the amplified signals, usually into either a visual or an auditory format that is easily understood by the individual. The third step is to provide real time information of change. Individuals eventually learn to control these physiological reactions by use of the real time feedback. For example, an athlete can sense the contraction state of his or her biceps with an EMG signal. Individuals can also have a sense of his or her physiological state through HR or EEG feedback. The main purpose of these processes is to assist the individual in increasing self-awareness through biofeedback information. According to the assumption of biofeedback, if individuals can sense and change information obtained from a specific physiological process, then they can learn to regulate the process. Therefore, an individual will be able to control a specific physiological process so long as the skill of control is sufficiently practiced (Andreassi, 1995).

Olson (1987) derived three theoretical models for biofeedback training: the Learning Theory Model, the Cybernetics Model, and the Stress Management Model. The focus of these models is varied, and none of them is comprehensive enough to be an independent system. The Learning Theory Model maintains that biofeedback training is the result of operational conditioning between neuromuscular and autonomic activity (e.g., muscle tension and HR results from the manipulation of behavioral control). The Cybernetics Model proposes that the devices and signals of biofeedback are the sources of information for the completion of the external feedback loop. Individuals will regulate or control their physiological process when they receive information that their physiological states (rest, stress, or relaxed) deviate. The Stress Management Model describes biofeedback as a noninvasive technique that helps individuals enhance their capacity for coping with stress.

General Application in Research

Biofeedback is a technique for self-regulation (Demos, 2005). It helps individuals learn control of physiological processes with the aid of a biofeedback device. In order to detect biological signals such as muscle, sweat, body temperature, and HR, sensors are attached to a specific part of body. Biological signals provided by the device help participants gain control of their mind through subconscious biological processes. Participants perceive a change in their physiological process of a specific body part at any given time through the real time signals provided by the device. The feedback signal can be a tone of an auditory modality in digital or analog format, or in visual form on a computer screen. The feedback signal helps participants to practice self-regulation.

Sport psychologists have been applying the concept of biofeedback training to assist athletes regulating their level of arousal since early 1980 (Zaichkowsky, 1983). Biofeedback training is usually used to enhance sport performance by helping athletes handle general and specific anxiety, reduce pain and fatigue, and enhance their adaptation (Blumenstein, 2002). In sports, the modality of biofeedback training includes EMG muscle feedback, skin thermometer feedback, galvanic skin response (GSR) feedback, EEG feedback, EKG and HR feedback, and blood pressure feedback. Among these modalities, EMG, GSR, HR, and EEG have been widely used for psychoregulation in recent years to enhance sport performance (Blumenstein, 2002). In a review, Zaichkowsky and Fuchs (1988) concluded that 60% of studies found EMG biofeedback training has a positive effect on sport performance. Petruzzello, Landers, and Salazar (1991) and Collins (1995) also concluded that HR, respiration, and EEG slow wave biofeedback training can enhance sport performance.

Neurofeedback Training and Sport Performance

Definition of Neurofeedback Training

Since it was first discovered and recorded, EEG has become a test tool for pathological diagnosis in clinical medicine. Kamiya (1969), a brain scientist from Chicago, asked participants to control their EEG at a certain frequency band. He found that it was possible to control EEG through learning. The frequently studied EEG frequencies in neurofeedback training include θ (4-8Hz), α (8-13Hz), β (13-20Hz), and Sensory Motor Rhythm (SMR; 12-15Hz). Studies suggest that θ is related to working memory (Burgess, & Gruzelier, 1997). Theta increases when the brain is encoding new information and retrieving information from long-term memory (Klimesch, 1999). Alpha is related to a relaxed but attentive state. Sensory stimulation and increase in mental activity is associated with inhibition of α activity. Surwillo (1963) found that α is related to the speed of information processing. Furthermore, α has been said to maintain and control the internal homeostasis of the cortex. In contrast to α and θ, β has been less studied.

An increase in β within the brain has been associated with attention and motor preparation. When attention load increases, β also increases (Steriade, 1993). SMR is also a less studied frequency. The psychophysiological significance of SMR is still not yet fully understood. Roth, Sterman, and Clemente (1967) found that when subjects inhibit limb movement, EEG activity appears in the 12-16 Hz frequency band. This EEG frequency is thus related to the brain's behavioral inhibition system.

EEG biofeedback is usually called neurofeedback. Neurofeedback mainly utilizes knowledge from neural anatomy, neurophysiology, and cognitive neuroscience for designing training methods to enhance brain function. Specifically, neurofeedback helps individuals gain control of their brain waves through the training of specific frequencies at specified electrodes. Usually, the training is aimed at enhancing the capacity of concentration, arousal control, and self-regulation. EEG recorded on an electrode mainly reflects the neural activity underlying that specified electrode. The concept of neurofeedback is based on the relationship between EEG activity of a specific frequency at a specified electrode and cognitive process or behavior. An EEG feature can be identified for stimulating or inhibiting neural activity that leads to control and regulates brain function. Neurofeedback has been used clinically to treat epilepsy (Sterman, 2000), attention deficit and hyperactivity disorder (ADHD; Lubar, & Lubar, 1999), alcohol addiction (Peniston, & Kulkosky, 1999), and posttraumatic stress disorder (Peniston, & Kulkosky), by improving the brain's self-regulation during the early stages of disease.

The brain is the control center of the human body, coordinating its thoughts, peripheral sensation, and motor systems, just like the central processing unit of a computer. Consequently, brain efficiency is closely related to sport performance. Blumenstein, Bar-Eli, and Tenenbaum (1997) proposed the Wingate five-step training to progressively guide participants into a neurofeedback program that would result in the best outcome. The first stage is introduction. Before the training starts, the researcher informs participants about the training process and key points that need their attention. The second stage is identification. Before designing the neurofeedback training protocol, the EEG features of a specific cognitive process have to be identified. The training protocol is then finalized after considering the connection between EEG features and behavior. The third stage is simulation. Neurofeedback training starts after the training protocol is identified. Participants try to control their brain waves to meet the criteria. Researchers modify the time and intensity of EEG control according to the individual's progress. The fourth stage is transformation. Participants start to apply the cognitive skills they learned through neurofeedback training to the real situation as soon as they have gained control of their EEG. The level of difficulty of situations for transformation is based on the participants' progress. The fifth stage is realization. At this stage, participants are able to progressively self-monitor their EEG activity without the assistance of an EEG machine. They can effectively apply the self-regulation into real-life situations such as during training and in competition.

Neurofeedback Training and Sport Performance

Since Hatfield et al.'s seminal paper (Hatfield, Landers, & Ray, 1984) found an increase in α power in the left temporal region (T3) of the brain when expert shooters approached trigger pull, a series of studies have explored the relationship between EEG and sport performance. Researchers have found that T3-α power is positively correlated with air pistol shooting performance (Loze, Collins, & Holmes, 2001) and the level of shooting skill (Haufler, Spalding, Santa Maria, & Hatfield, 2000). The T3-α finding is interpreted as being due to the hemispheric specialization of the brain. Shooting is considered a visuo-spatial task that is more specialized in the right side of the brain, while the left side is more involved in the verbal-analytical process. The progressive increase at T3-α while expert shooters approach trigger pull implies an inhibition of the left temporal brain activation that is related to a verbal-analytical process deemed less relevant to the shooting task. If this mechanistic interpretation holds, an increase in T3-α through neurofeedback training should enhance shooting performance. Despite calling for such a study by some researchers (e.g., Vernon, 2005), up to now, only a few studies have examined this possibility. Landers and his colleagues (1991) conducted the first study of this kind. The authors assigned pre-elite archers into three groups. The "correct neurofeedback" group received one session of 45-75 minutes of neurofeedback training aimed at enhancing left temporal low frequency EEG. The "incorrect neurofeedback" group received the same duration of neurofeedback training to enhance the low frequency EEG at the right temporal region of the brain. The "control" group received no treatment. Results showed

that archery performance in the "correct neurofeedback" group was significantly better than that in the two other groups, and in the "incorrect neurofeedback" group archery performance was lower. However, there was no statistical difference in EEG activity among these three groups. An explanation for the lack of variation in EEG activity is that only one session of neurofeedback training was employed. Improving upon this study by providing more training sessions, Lin (2007) applied neurofeedback training to a small group of skilled archers. Compared to the control group that received no training sessions (N = 5), the neurofeedback group (N = 6) received three sessions of neurofeedback training each week for two weeks. Each session of training lasted for about 20-25 minutes. Alpha at T3 was deducted by T4 to derive a lateralization index. The author found that (1) archery performance in the neurofeedback group at post-training was better than at pre-training; (2) there was no difference in alpha lateralization at post-training between groups; (3) there was a trend but no statistical difference of higher T3-α and β in post-training than in pre-training in the neurofeedback group. Lin suggested that more training sessions may make a difference.

Recently, Wang and Hung (2006) found that neurofeedback training at T3-α in skilled air pistol shooters successfully enhanced shooting performance. Most importantly, the training also significantly increased T3-α. Neither shooting performance nor T3-α changed in the control group. These findings are encouraging because this is the first study showing covariation between T3-α and sport performance as a result of neurofeedback training. The authors attributed the findings to a high number of training sessions (i.e., 16 sessions over a duration of 6 weeks) and a systematic protocol for the neurofeedback training. As reported by the authors, the criterion of T3-α power was individually determined. The training was first held in the lab and then gradually moved into the field.

Neurofeedback training has also been used to enhance dance performance. Raymond, Sajid, Parkinson, and Gruzelier (2005) compared the effects of neurofeedback and HR biofeedback training on dance performance. The neurofeedback training employed the α/θ model for 10 sessions over a period of four weeks, each session lasting for 20 minutes. The results showed that both types of training can effectively enhance dance performance. Neurofeedback training was more effective in improving dance tempo than was HR biofeedback training. The authors attributed the improvement of dance tempo performance to the reduction of anxiety.

Mechanism of the Effects of Neurofeedback Training on Enhancing Sport Performance

How neurofeedback training enhances sport performance requires further investigation. Three possible explanations are discussed here.

(1) Optimizing Levels of Arousal

Arousal is a continuum from deep sleep to extreme excitement. Changes in levels of arousal are usually associated with increased/decreased activation in the sympathetic and the parasympathetic nervous system. Research in sport psychology has indicated that in some circumstances, elevated arousal is associated with the induction of negative emotions such as anxiety and tension. Sport psychologists claim a close relationship between level of arousal and sport performance. Theories such as the inverted U hypothesis and individual zone of optimal functioning presume that optimal arousal regulation is a prerequisite for peak performance. The EEG frequency neurofeedback-targeted training is usually based on its relation to specific mental states. For instance, α is related to a state of attentiveness, consciousness, calmness, and homeostasis of the brain (Ray, 1990). Elevation of arousal accompanies inhibition of α (Davidson & Irwin, 1999). This is because the level of arousal affects oscillation of the brain (Newman, 1995; Robinson, 2002). This view is consistent with Elul's (1972) hypothesis of EEG genesis, in which it is theorized that the thalamus is the pacemaker of the brain's sensory-perception process and the thalamo-cortical pathway is related to α activity. The thalamus is located in the center of the limbic system. It receives input from modalities of the peripheral sensory neurons and provides output to the relevant cortex. Change in EEG activity in the cortex is a result of regulation in sensory information by the thalamus. This view is supported by neuroscience findings that brain-originated self-regulation disorders are related to the thalamus. Lately, neuroscientists have speculated that the hypothalamus in the limbic system is related to homeostasis (e.g., body temperature and endocrine) and arousal regulation.

The view that the performance enhancement effect of neurofeedback training occurs through arousal regulation is corroborated by Chang, Wang, and Hung's (2007) study, which reports that T3-α neurofeedback training enhances α not only at T3 but also in other regions. This general elevation of α across a wide cortical region indicates that neurofeedback training has lowered arousal—conducive to performance in sports such as shooting, in which a lower level of arousal is considered beneficial.

(2) Attention Control

Hatfield and Hillman's (2001) Psychomotor Efficiency Hypothesis suggests that skilled sport performance is characterized by the allocation of neural resources in such a way that the activity of nonessential neural processes is reduced. This hypothesis implies that a decrease in interference from these nonessential neural processes to the essential neural network responsible for the sport task is key to performance enhancement. Thus, a reduction in interference from nonessential processes to the essential processes is an indication of concentration. One common assumption is that the left temporal region (i.e., T3) is a cortical area more involved in the verbal-analytical process, which is considered less relevant for a right-handed skilled shooter/archer. As such, in these studies the goal of neurofeedback training was to increase alpha activity in the left temporal region. Based on the "cortical idling" interpretation of EEG alpha power (Pfurtscheller, 1992), an increase of alpha power in the left temporal region is an indication of reduced verbal-analytical processes. Thus the participants can better concentrate on the shooting/archery task, which is more visuo-spatial in nature. In a similar vein, researchers have shown higher theta activity at the frontal region of the brain in children with ADHD (Chabot & Serfontein, 1996). Neurofeedback training chooses the beta band in the frontal region to activate the neural activity in this area of the brain because beta is associated with excitement.

(3) Change in Neurotransmitter Activity

Neurotransmitters play a critical role in neural communication. The levels of neurotransmitters affect the efficacy of information processing and homeostasis of the brain. A shortage or oversupply of neurotransmitters results in abnormal cognitive function and behavior. As a result, maintaining a normal level of neurotransmitters is crucial to normal function of the brain. For example, persons with a deficiency in their attention system are prescribed Ritalin, a medicine that regulates neurotransmitters, to improve attention function. Research has shown higher theta activity in ADHD children (Chabot & Serfontein, 1996). Rossieter and LaVaque (1995) found that after three months of intervention, both the neurofeedback training group and the Ritalin medication group improved in attention performance. Another study found similar results (Monastra, Monastra, & George, 2002). These studies showed that neurofeedback could be as effective as medication. Moreover, there have been no side effects reported in neurofeedback studies. More evidence supporting the neurotransmitter hypothesis comes from Egner and Gruzelier (2001). They found that the amplitude of P300, a component of event-related potentials, increases significantly after neurofeedback training. The amplitude of P300 has been associated with attention resource. The enhancement of P300 amplitude after neurofeedback training indicates that participants were able to allocate more attention resources to process information. Some researchers assume that as both the frequency of stimulation to the brain and the amount of motor practices increase, the connection between neurons will be strengthened. The efficient release of neurotransmitters and better functioning of the synapses facilitate the communication between neurons (Classen, Lippert, Wise, Hallet, & Cohen, 1998). The therapeutic effect of neurofeedback training has been applied in clinical settings for patients with attention deficiency (Kropotov et al., 2005) and emotional disorders (Raymond et al., 2005). Generally, these studies found significant positive effects from neurofeedback training. Because the patients usually suffered from a neurotransmitter disorder, the effect of neurofeedback training must have something to do with the alteration of neurotransmitters. Kotchoubey et al. (1999) and Kropotov et al. (2005) pointed out that the main function of neurofeedback training is either to stimulate or inhibit neural activity at certain cortical regions. The training can regulate release of neurotransmitters and improve the regulation capacity of the nervous system. However, there are no studies to verify this hypothesis that directly measure the change of neurotransmitters as a result of neurofeedback training.

Heart Rate Feedback and Sport Performance

Attention always plays an important role in sport performance. For example, coaches will ask athletes to clear their minds during competition and try not to be dis-turbed by noise from the surrounding environment. Research has shown that concentration in games and the use of narrow attention are critical for athletes to achieve peak performance (Ravizza, 1977). HR has been considered an interesting index with potential application among the factors influencing attention.

Link between Heart Rate and Attention

The theoretic basis of association between HR and attention was first elucidated by Lacey's intake-reject hypothesis (Lacey, 1967). It was considered that the deceleration of HR is related to the intake of stimuli and information from the external environment, and conversely, the acceleration of HR is related to the rejection of stimuli and information from the external environment. Based on this hypothesis, the deceleration of HR occurs when individual attention is directed by information from external environments whereas the acceleration of HR takes place if individual attention is focused more on the self than externally. The visceral afferent feedback model later developed by Lacey and Lacey (1974, 1980) theorizes that the individual HR will slow down when the individual is paying attention to something external. This weakens the inhibitions from the autonomic nervous system to the medulla and strengthens the process of receiving external stimuli. In contrast, when individuals focus on themselves or perform self-talk, their HR speeds up because the inhibitions from the autonomic nervous system to the medulla are strengthened. The individual internal cognition processes external stimuli as a "noise," and forms a block to stop the reception of stimuli as well as information from the outside environment. The intake-reject hypothesis seems to be more complete if it is combined with the model of visceral afferent feedback. In his article "Mind your Heart," Carlstedt (2001) regards changes of HR as a reflection of how individuals make use of their attention. When people pay attention to a specific event in the surrounding environment or individual attention is directed internally, the HR will decelerate or accelerate, respectively.

Research has shown results to support the aforementioned hypothesis. Lacey and Lacey (1970) found that participants' HR decreased 3-4 times between cue and execution signals in reaction time experiments. This phenomenon was ascribed to participants' attention to pictures on the computer monitor; the change of attention caused the HR change. Stern (1976) found an association between attention and HR change in the 5-second interval between "Get ready" and "Go" in cycling and sprinting. The acceleration of HR was observed the 5 seconds before the "Go" signal, whereas the deceleration appeared in the second just prior to the "Go" signal. The decrease of HR was significant in the second before the athletes began to run, due to their focus on the signal "Go." Both studies support the association between attention and HR change provided by Lacey's intake-reject hypothesis as well as by Lacey and Lacey's visceral afferent feedback model.

Heart Rate and Sport Performance

As to the relation between motor performance and HR change, some studies have investigated the association between precision sports and deceleration of HR. In a study involving 17 elite rifle shooters, Hatfield, Landers, and Ray (1987) found that participants showed an acceleration of HR in the stage of aiming (i.e., 2.5-5 seconds prior to trigger pull), whereas a deceleration of HR was observed when approaching trigger pull. Salazar et al. (1990) observed similar results in an archery study: Participants showed an increase of 3-4 seconds in HR prior to the release of the arrow. HR decreased when approaching arrow release. Additionally, when archers drew the bow fully and paid attention to the target, their HR was slower than when they were relaxed. Landers et al. (1994) observed significant deceleration of HR in the period between aiming and arrow release; their results supported Salazar's (1990) finding. These authors interpret the phenomena of HR deceleration as a reflection of how the archers and rifle shooters were eliminating any thoughts in their mind (e.g., self-talk and worries) and placing their attention solely on aiming at the target. The HR deceleration can strengthen the athletes' ability to receive information provided by the external environment so that they can be relaxed and steady when using motor skills.

After understanding the association between HR and attention, it is pertinent to discuss the association between change of HR and sport performance. Tremayne and Barry (2001) separated participants into two groups in order to study the relationship between shooting performance and HR deceleration. The experimental groups included 10 players who were elite shooters and the control group contained 10 novices. Results showed that the level of performance was related to HR deceleration for elite shooters in the period of 5

seconds prior to trigger pull. A significant deceleration of HR was observed in high shooting scores (i.e., good performance), whereas there was no significant HR change in poor performance. Furthermore, HR deceleration occurred at 3.5 seconds prior to trigger pull in good performance. In addition to performance, the level of HR deceleration varied in relation to the player's skill level. Studies have found that elite players have higher degrees of HR deceleration than do novices, who usually show small or insignificant degrees of HR deceleration. Molander and Backman (1989) found that 6 golfers who were 30 years old showed significant deceleration of HR during training and the trend became more obvious as training continued. The association between poor performance and acceleration of HR was also observed in six 50-year-old golfers.

Similarly, Boutcher and Zinsser (1990) found that the HR of elite golfers decreased 4-11 beats per minute during the 3-7 seconds prior to golf putt. Based on the results of this and the above studies, the performance of precision sport and the skill level of players seem to be related to HR change. According to the intake-reject hypothesis and the visceral afferent feedback model (Lacey 1967; Lacey & Lacey 1974, 1980), good performance is associated with higher degrees of HR deceleration. This is because more external attention is designated for target aiming in order to strengthen the process of receiving information from the surrounding environment. Thus, the elite shooters are able to pull the trigger more precisely. In contrast, the phenomenon of HR deceleration is not significantly shown in poor performance because participants are not able to change their direction of attention. A recent study on intermediate shooters found a significant difference between good and poor performance according to the deceleration of HR. Similar to previous studies, good performance showed a systematic deceleration of HR, whereas in poor performance no HR deceleration could be observed. If the precision athletes are able to maintain an appropriate direction of attention, the deceleration of HR will be more obvious and shooting performance will be enhanced (Liu, Liu, Shih, & Hung, 2006).

After establishing the association between HR deceleration and precision sport performance, the logical next step is to develop methods that can facilitate athletes' HR deceleration. Green, Green, and Walters (1970) believe that every physiological reaction in the body is accompanied by mental or emotional change.

Similarly, every mental or emotional change will affect physiological reaction. The use of biofeedback training to control physiological reactions (e.g., reduce performance anxiety, increase muscle strength, reduce pain and fatigue, regulate HR, and enhance attention) is a legitimate approach to enhancing sport performance (Chen & Lu, 2003). Research has shown that using biofeedback training to induce relaxation response can effectively reduce HR, stress reactivity, and coping response in archers (Shen, 1993). In another study, Huang (1994) found that combined with relaxation and imagery training, biofeedback training can enhance putting performance and self-report psychological skills, as well as reduce HR and blood pressure in elite golfers. Blumenstein, Breslav, Bar-Eli, Tenenbaum, and Weinstein (1995) found that both HR and blood pressure dropped, and sport performance also improved, when biofeedback training was used to induce relaxation response. Lin (2007) conducted a study of HR deceleration training and sport performance among archers. In his report, skilled archers were separated into either the biofeedback group (BF) or the control group (CO). In addition to routine training, the BF underwent 16 sessions of HR biofeedback training lasting a period of 5 weeks. In contrast, the CO received "faked" HR biofeedback training. The faked training was designed to prevent the CO from incurring any psychological effects resulting from being in a control group. Results showed that both archery performance and HR deceleration improved significantly in the BF, but neither of these was observed in the CO. This study provides evidence for facilitating HR deceleration through biofeedback training, and offers another approach to practitioners for applying mental regulation in performance enhancement.

Conclusion

Advancements in psychophysiology and cognitive neuroscience clearly show the close relationship between body and mind. Biofeedback training is an application of this close body-mind connection. Although the discussion of biofeedback training is limited to EEG and HR in this chapter, the intention was to show the great potential of biofeedback in fostering an understanding of how the mind works. In sports, both neurofeedback and HR biofeedback have been used in self-regulation with some success. Although the studies reviewed in this chapter illustrate the validity of biofeedback training in performance enhancement, it is still quite puzzling as to how little research has been done in this area. One reason that explains the limited amount of study in this area could be the barrier to acquiring and using electronic devices. However, with the rapid development of electronics, the cost of a typical biofeedback device is currently inexpensive and the operation has become much more user-friendly. Finally, collaboration among researchers with different kinds of expertise is required to overcome equipment and technical difficulties. These developments could provide momentum to future studies on this subject.

References

Andreassi, J. L. (1995). *Psychophysiology: Human behavior and physical response* (3rd ed.). Hillsdale, NJ: Erlbaum.

Basmajian, J. V. (Ed.). (1978). *Biofeedback: Principles and practice for clinicians.* Baltimore: Williams & Wilkins.

Blanchard, E. B., & Goodstein, L. H. (1978). *A biofeedback primer.* Reading, MA: Addison-Wesley.

Blumenstein, B. (2002). Biofeedback applications in sport and exercise: Research findings. In B. Blumenstein, M. Bar-Eli, & G. Tenenbaum (Eds.), *Brain and body in sport and exercise: Biofeedback applications in performance enhancement* (pp. 37-54). New York: Wiley.

Blumenstein, B., Bar-Eli, M., & Tenenbaum, G. (1997). A five-step approach to mental training incorporating biofeedback. *The Sport Psychologist, 11,* 440-453.

Blumenstein, B., Breslav, I., Bar-Eli, M., Tenenbaum, G., & Weinstein, Y. (1995). Regulation of mental states and biofeedback techniques: Effects on breathing patterns. *Biofeedback and Self-regulation, 20,* 169-183.

Boutcher, S. H. (1992). Attention and athletic performance: An integrated approach. In T. S. Horn (Ed.), *Advances in sport psychology* (pp. 251-266). Champaign, IL: Human Kinetics.

Boutcher, S. H., & Zinsser, N. W. (1990). Cardiac deceleration of elite and beginning golfers during putting. *Journal of Sport and Exercise Psychology, 12,* 37-47.

Burgess, A. P., & Gruzelier, J. H. (1997). Short duration of synchronization of human theta rhythm during recognition memory. *Neuroreport, 8,* 1039-1042.

Carlstedt, R. A. (2001, August). Mind your heart. *The Journal of the American Board of Sport Psychology* (On-Line Journal). Retrieved November 20, 2006, from http://www.americanboardofsportpsychology.org/Portals/24/MindYourHeart.pdf.

Chabot, R. T., & Serfontein, G. (1996). Sensitivity and specificity of QEEG in children with attention deficit or specific developmental learning disorders. *Biological Psychiatry, 40,* 951-963.

Chang, T., Wang, Y., & Hung, T. (2007, September). *Neurofeedback training enhances α power.* Paper presented at the annual meeting of the European Federation for Sport Psychology, Halkidiki, Greece.

Chen, L., & Lu, J. (2003). Effect of biofeedback training to sport performance. *College Physical Education, 68,* 165-171. (Chinese)

Classen, J., Lippert, J., Wise, S. P., Hallet, M., & Cohen, L. G. (1998). Rapid plasticity of human cortical movement representation induced by practice. *Journal of Neurophysiology, 79*, 1117-1123.

Collins, D. (1995). Psychophysiology and sport performance. In S. J. H. Biddle (Ed.), *European perspectives on exercise and sport psychology* (pp. 154-178). Champaign, IL: Human Kinetics.

Davidson, R. J., & Irwin, W. (1999). The functional neuroanatomy of emotion and affective style. *Trends in Cognitive Science, 3*, 11-21.

Demos, J. N. (2005). *Getting started with neurofeedback*. New York: W. W. Norton & Company.

Egner, T., & Gruzelier, J. H. (2001). Learned self-regulation of EEG frequency components affects attention and even-related brain potentials in humans. *NeuroReport, 12*, 4155-4160.

Elul, R. (1972). Randomness and synchrony in the generation of the electroencephalogram. In H. Petsche & M. A. B. Brazier (Eds.), *Synchronization of EEG activity in epilepsies* (pp. 59-77). Vienna: Springer Verlag.

Feltz, D. L. (1984). Self-efficacy as a cognitive mediator of athletic performance. In W. F. Straup & J. M. Williams (Eds.), *Cognitive sport psychology* (pp. 191-198). Lansing, NY: Sport Science Associates.

Fitts, P. M., & Posner, M. I. (1967). *Human performance*. Belmont, CA: Brooks/Cole.

Green, E., Green, A., & Walters, D. (1970). Voluntary control of internal states: Psychological and physiological. *Journal of Transpersonal Psychology, 1*, 2-26.

Hatfield, B. D., & Hillman, C. H. (2001). The psychophysiology of sport: A mechanistic understanding of the psychology of superior performance. In R. Singer, H. Hausenblas, & C. Janelle (Eds.), *Handbook of sport psychology* (pp. 362-386). New York: Wiley.

Hatfield, B. D., Landers, D. M., & Ray, W. J. (1984). Cognitive processes during self-paced motor performance: An electroencephalographic profile of skilled marksmen. *Journal of Sport Psychology, 6*, 42-59.

Hatfield, B. D., Landers, D. M., & Ray, W. J. (1987). Cardiovascular-CNS interactions during a self-paced, intentional attentive state: Elite marksmanship performance. *Psychophysiology, 24*, 542-549.

Haufler, A. J., Spalding, T. W., Santa Maria, D. L., & Hatfield, B. D. (2000). Neuro-cognitive activity during a self-paced visuo-spatial task: Comparative EEG profiles in marksmen and novice shooters. *Biological Psychology, 53*, 131-160.

Huang, C. (1994). Effects of biofeedback training, progressive muscle relaxation, and imagery training on coping in stress and sport performance in elite athletes. In J. Wang & L. Chi (Eds.), *Thesis in Sport Psychology: Vol. 2.* (pp. 453-474). Taipei: Psychology Publisher. (Chinese)

Kamiya, J. (1969). Operant control of the EEG alpha rhythm and some of its reported effects on consciousness. In C. T. Tart (Ed.), *Altered states of consciousness* (pp. 507-517). New York: Wiley.

Klimesch, W. (1999). EEG alpha and theta oscillations reflect cognitive and memory performance: A review and analysis. *Brain Research Review, 29*, 169-195.

Kotchoubey, B., Busch, S., Strehl, U., & Birbaumer, N. (1999). Changes in EEG power spectra during biofeedback of slow cortical potentials in epilepsy. *Applied Psychophysiology and Biofeedback, 24*, 213-233.

Kropotov, J. D., Grin-Yatsenko, V. A., Ponomarev, V. A., Chutko, L. S., Yakovenko, E. A., & Nikishena, I. S. (2005). ERPs correlates of EEG relative beta training in ADHD children. *International Journal of Psychophysiology, 55*, 23-34.

Lacey, B. C., & Lacey, J. I. (1970). Some autonomic-central nervous system interrelationship. In P. Black (Ed.), *Physiological correlates of emotion* (pp. 205-228). New York: Academic Press.

Lacey, B. C., & Lacey, J. I. (1974). Studies of HR and other bodily processes in sensorimotor behavior. In P. A. Obrist, A. H. Black, J. Brener, & L. V. DiCara (Eds.), *Cardiovascular psychophysiology* (pp. 538-564). Chicago: Aldine.

Lacey, B. C., & Lacey, J. I. (1980). Cognitive modulation of time-dependent primary bradycardia. *Psychophysiology, 17*, 209-221.

Lacey, J. I. (1967). Somatic response patterning and stress: Some revisions of activation theory. In M. H. Appley & R. Trumbull (Eds.), *Psychological stress* (pp. 14-42). New York: Appleton-Century Croft.

Landers, D. M. (1980). The arousal-performance relationship revisited. *Research Quarterly for Exercise and Sport, 51*, 77-90.

Landers, D. M., Han, M., Salazar, W., Petruzzello, S., Kubitz, K., & Gannon, T. (1994). Effects of learning on electroencephalographic and electrocardiographic patterns in novice archers. *International Journal of Sport Psychology, 25*, 56-70.

Landers, D. M., Petruzzello, S. J., Salazar, W., Crews, D. J., Kubitz, K. A., Gannon, T. L., et al. (1991). The influence of electrocortical biofeedback on performance in pre-elite archers. *Medicine and Science in Sport and Exercise, 23*, 123-128.

Lin, P. (2007). *The effects of biofeedback training on HR activity of archers*. Unpublished master's thesis, Taipei Physical Education College, Taipei.

Lin, P. Y., Lin, J. H., Shih, H. S., & Hung, T. M. (2006, June). *HR deceleration is associated with better performance in intermediate air pistol shooters*. Paper presented at the annual meeting of the North American Society for Psychology of Sport and Physical Activity, Denver, CO.

Loze, G. M., Collins, D., & Holmes, P. S. (2001). Pre-shot EEG alpha-power during expert air-pistol shooting: A comparison of best and worst shot. *Journal of Sports Sciences, 19*, 727-733.

Lubar, J. F., & Lubar, J. O. (1999). Neurofeedback assessment and treatment for attention deficit/hyperactive disorder. In J. R. Evans & A. Arbarbanel (Eds.), *Introduction to quantitative EEG and neurofeedback* (pp. 103-143). San Diego, CA: Academic Press.

Meichenbaum, D. H. (1977). *Cognitive-behavior modification: An integrative approach*. New York: Plenum Press.

Molander, B., & Backman, L. (1989). Age differences in HR patterns during concentration in a precision sport: Implications for attentional functioning. *Journal of Gerontology, 44*, 80-87.

Monastra, V. J., Monastra, D. M., & George, S. (2002). The effects of stimulant therapy, EEG biofeedback, and parenting style on the primary symptoms of attention-deficit/hyperactivity disorder. *Applied Psychophysiology and Biofeedback, 27*, 231–249.

Moss, D. (1994). *Twenty-fifth anniversary yearbook*. Wheat Ridge, CO; Association for Applied Psychophysiology and Biofeedback.

Newman, J. (1995). Thalamic contributions to attention and consciousness. *Consciousness and Cognition, 4*, 172-193.

Olson, R. P. (1987). Definitions of biofeedback and applied psychophysiology. In M. S. Schwartz, & Associates (Eds.), *Biofeedback: A practitioner's guide* (pp. 27-31). New York: Guilford Press.

Peniston, E. G., & Kulkosky, P. J. (1999). Neurofeedback in the treatment of addictive disorder. In J. R. Evans & A. Arbarbanel

(Eds.), *Introduction to quantitative EEG and neurofeedback* (pp. 157-179). San Diego, CA: Academic Press.

Petruzzello, S. J., Landers, D. M., & Salazar, W. (1991). Biofeedback and sport/exercise performance: Applications and limitations. *Behavior Therapy, 22,* 379-392.

Pfurtscheller, G. (1992). Event-related synchronization (ERS): An electrophysiological correlate of cortical areas at rest. *Electroencephalography and Clinical Neurophysiology, 83,* 62-69.

Ravizza, K. (1977). Peak experience in sport. *Journal of Humanistic Psychology, 17,* 35-40.

Ray, W. J. (1990). The electrocortical system. In J. T. Cacioppo & L. G. Tassinary (Eds.), *Principles of psychophysiology* (pp. 385-412). Cambridge, England: Cambridge University Press.

Ray, W. J., Raczynski, J. M., Rogers, T., & Kimball, W. H. (1979). *Evaluation of clinical biofeedback.* New York: Plenum Press.

Raymond, J., Sajid I., Parkinson, L. A., & Gruzelier, J. H. (2005). Biofeedback and dance performance: A preliminary investigation. *Applied Psychophysiology and Biofeedback, 30,* 65-73.

Robazza, C., Bortoli, L., & Nougier, V. (2000). Performance emotions in an elite archer: A case study. *Journal of Sport Behavior, 23,* 144-163.

Robinson, D. L. (2002). How brain arousal systems determine different temperament types and major dimensions of personality. *Personality and Individual Differences, 28,* 673-693.

Rossieter, T. R., & LaVaque, T. J. (1995). A comparison of EEG biofeedback and psychostimulants in treating attention deficit/hyperactivity disorders. *Journal of Neurotherapy, 1,* 48–59.

Roth, S. R., Sterman, M. B., & Clemente, C. D. (1967). Comparison of EEG correlates of reinforcement, internal inhibition and sleep. *Electroencephalography and Clinical Neurophysiology, 23,* 509-520.

Salazar, W., Landers, D. M., Petruzzello, S. J., Han, M. W., Crews, D. J., & Kubitz, K. A. (1990). Hemispheric asymmetry, cardiac response, and performance in elite archers. *Research Quarterly for Exercise and Sport, 61,* 351-359.

Schwartz, G. E., & Beatty, J. (1977). *Biofeedback: Theory and research.* New York: Academic Press.

Shen, L. (1993). Effects of relaxation training, biofeedback training, and imagery training on coping in stress of the elite archers. In J. Wang & L. Chi (Eds.), *Thesis in sport psychology: Vol. 1* (pp. 277-300). Taipei: Psychology Publisher. (Chinese)

Steriade M. (1993). Cellular substrates of brain rhythms. In E. Niedermeyer & F. Lopes de Silva (Eds.), *Electroencephalography: Basic principles, clinical applications, and related fields* (pp. 27-62). Baltimore: Williams and Wilkins.

Sterman, M. B. (2000). Basic concept of clinical findings in the treatment of seizure disorders with EEG operant conditioning. *Clinical Electroencephalography, 31,* 45-55.

Stern, R. (1976). Reaction time and HR between the GET SET and GO of simulated races. *Psychophysiology, 13,* 149-154.

Surwillo, W. W. (1963). The relation of simple response time to brain-wave frequency and the effects of age. *Electroencephalography and Clinical Neurophysiology, 15,* 105.

Tremayne, P., & Barry, R. J. (2001). Elite pistol shooters: Physiological patterning of best vs. worst shots. *International Journal of Psychophysiology, 41,* 19-29.

Vernon, D. J. (2005). Can neurofeedback training enhance performance? An evaluation of the evidence with implications for future research. *Applied Psychophysiology and Biofeedback, 30,* 347-364.

Wang, Y., & Hung, T. (2006, October). *Effects of neurofeedback training on EEG and shooting performance.* Paper presented at the annual meeting of the Chinese Association of Sport Psychology, Wuhan, China.

Weinberg, R. S., & Gould, D. (2007). *Foundations of sport and exercise psychology* (4th ed). Champaign, IL: Human Kinetics.

Zaichkowsky, L. D. (1983). The use of biofeedback for self-regulation of performance states. In L. E. Unestahl (Ed.), *The mental aspects of gymnastics* (pp. 95-105). Örebro, Sweden: Veje.

Zaichkowsky, L. D., & Fuchs, C. Z. (1988). Biofeedback applications in exercise and athletic performance. In K. B. Pandolf (Ed.), *Exercise and sport sciences reviews* (pp. 381-421). New York: Macmillan.

CHAPTER 13

Integrating the Eastern Martial Arts' *Chi* Concept into Psychological Skills Training

FRANK J. H. LU

Chi is an eastern martial arts' concept which, by its simplest definition, represents one's life vital force. However, there is more than vital force in martial artists' conceptualization of *Chi* when they use it as a tool to promote health or enhance power, or even to control anxiety while performing. Because the practice of *Chi* is similar to the practice of psychological skills training (PST), the purpose of this chapter is to introduce this concept for sport psychologists. To achieve this end, this issue is addressed in four parts. First, I will briefly introduce the concept of *Chi*. Second, I will address the link between *Chi* and PST. Third, I will present how to apply *Chi* in athletic settings. Finally, I will conclude the chapter, making a connection to sport excellence.

The Concept of *Chi*

What is *Chi*?

Chi is also known as *Ki* or *Qi*, depending on the pronunciation system used. Generally speaking, the Japanese and Koreans use *Ki* more often than *Chi* or *Qi*. In Chinese-language speaking areas such as Taiwan,

Hong Kong, Macau, and Singapore, they use *Chi* more often than *Qi*, which is used mostly in mainland China (http://www.balckbeltmag.com/archives/486). Recently, because of the economic and political boom in China, especially since Hong Kong and Macau have been returned to China, more people use *Qi* than *Chi* in their pronunciation.

By its simplest meaning, *Chi* is internal energy or life force energy, which is similar to the Greek "pneuma" and the Sanskrit "prana" of India. Eastern people believe that *Chi* is the vital force and energy flow in all living things (Yang, 1990). According to the Chinese dictionary, *Chi* also means *air*. The old Chinese saying, "there are three essentials in all lives—air, water, and sunshine," indicated the importance of air. Chinese herb doctors borrow this concept, combining the above mentioned vital force and energy concept; they argued that when illness is in a certain part of body, for example an old man's knee, it is because the *Chi* in that man is being stagnated so they use acupuncture or herbs to direct the *Chi*. Sometimes the word *Chi* is applied in a broader context, to refer to living and non-living subjects. For example, if one country is in a difficult situation of political or economic turbulence, one (mostly fortune tellers or astrologists) would describe this country's *Chi* as very weak. The Chinese *Fen-Sui* (geomancy) also borrows the concept of *Chi* in the identification of the location of buildings or houses. If the location of a building or house is good, which means bringing prosperity to the owner, the geomancer would say the location is full of *Chi*.

The concept of *Chi* began very early, around 4700 years ago, when a Chinese classical medicine book titled *Nei Ching Su Wen* [Classic Internal Medicine] described the relationship between illness and circulation of *Chi*. This book taught people to use either herbs or a sharp needle (i.e., today's acupuncture) to stimulate one's body, so as to enhance or facilitate the flow of *Chi* and cure illness. Evidence of using needles or sharp tools to stimulate *Chi* has been found in archaeological discoveries in Henan Province, China, where some stone probes called *Bian Shih* (stone needle) identified in the Shang dynasty (1766-1154 BC) provided evidence that people used tools to cure illness by stimulating the body's acupuncturing points (Choy, 1999; Connor, 1992; Huang, 1984; Yang, 1990).

According to *Chi-Far-Lun* [theory of *Chi*], *Chi* circulates throughout the human body along the *Gin* (channel) and *Lou* (sub-channels). The *Gin* and *Lou* cannot be seen by eyes but can be felt by stimulating the acupuncture points to identify them. According to *Chi-Far-Lun*, there are 12 main *Gins* which allow *Chi* to circulate throughout the whole body, connecting to major internal organs, nerves, or arteries. The 12 *Gins* govern the function of human internal organs, such as the heart, liver, gall bladder, spleen, stomach, and kidneys. Along the 12 *Gins* are many "cavities" where the acupuncture points are located, which connect to these organs, such as the heart, liver, gall bladder, spleen, stomach, and kidneys.

In addition, there are eight special *Meis* (vessels), which control the functioning of the nerves as well as endocrine secretion. Specifically, two major vessels, termed *Ren Mei* or Conception Vessel, which runs down the center of the body in front, and the *Du Mei* or Governing Vessel, which runs down the center of the back and the head, are particularly significant. When martial artists practice *Chi*, they imagine that the flow of *Chi* is along *Ren Mei* (a hypothetical central line on the anterior part of the body that starts from inside of the bladder and goes to the navel, chest, pharynx, chin,

mouth, nose, and to head) and *Du Mei* (a hypothetical central line on the posterior part of the body that starts from the sacrum and goes to the lumbar, shoulder, neck and back to the head), see Figure 1, which are believed to develop positive power or generate greater power for human functioning (Huang, 1984; Yang, 1990).

Chi and *Tai Chi Chuan*

Modern people's interest in the practice of *Chi* starts from a legendary Chinese martial arts Grand Master named San-Feng Chang, the founder of *Tai Chi Chuan*, in the Sung dynasty (AD 960-1297) San-Feng Chang used the theory of Chinese medicine to create *Tai Chi Chuan*, which is similar to western bare hand gymnastics but with a strong emphasis on the theory of *Chi*. *Tai Chi Chuan* has many schools based on San-Feng Chuan. The most famous school of *Tai Chi Chuan* is Wang-Ting Chen's' clan in the Ming and the beginning of the Ch'ing dynasty in China (Huang, 1984).

Chi and *Chi-Kung*

Also borrowing from the concept of Chinese medicine, the martial artists in China, Korea, and Japan created *Chi-Kung* [the works of Chi]. *Chi-Kung* is another style of affiliated martial arts. The major objective of practicing *Chi-Kung* is to enhance one's power of *Chi*. Every clan of martial arts schools in China, Korea, and Japan, whether it is Kung Fu, Taekwondo, Karate, Aikido, or Judo, claimed they were the originators of *Chi-Kung*. Although the inventor of *Chi-Kung* has never been identified, martial artists generally believe it is derived from San-Feng Chang's *Tai Chi Chuan*. Today, *Chi-Kung* is not only the principal method of practicing *Chi* for maintaining health, but is also an affiliate training for enhancing greater physical power because it facilitates martial artists' concentration, which, in turn, allows them to perform better than those who do not use *Chi-Kung* (Choy, 1999; Connor, 1992; Dunn, 1990; Lam, 2003; Yang, 1990).

The Practice of *Chi-Kung*

In general, regardless of which school of martial arts is followed, the practice of *Chi-Kung* includes four parts: (a) theory and philosophy, (b) exercise, (c) breathing, and, (d) meditation. The basic theory and philosophy have been presented in the introductory part of this chapter. As to the exercise of *Chi-Kung*, every school of martial arts has its own approach— from either San-

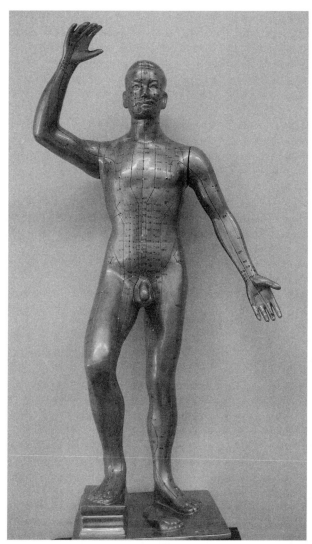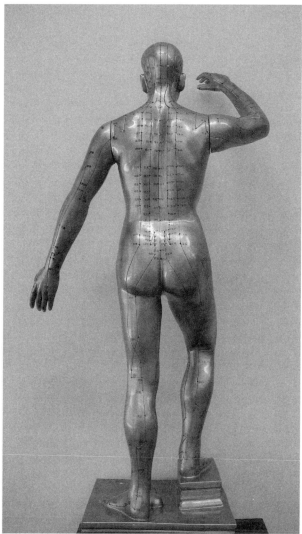

Figure 1

Feng Chang's *Tai Chi Chuan* or the ancient Chinese medical doctor Hua-Tor's (141-213 BC) Wu-Chin-Si (5 animal exercise), which imitates the movements of the tiger, deer, monkey, bear, and bird. A fundamental movement of *Chi's* exercise is performed by raising one's hands, twisting the trunk, stretching the limbs and trunk, or swinging the body. When performing these movements, controlled breathing is an essential element; in conjunction, those who practice *Chi* are told to imagine that the flow of *Chi* is circulating along the channels of *Gin* and *Lou*, respectively (Choy, 1999; Connor, 1992; Sun & Li, 1997; Yang, 1990).

Although there are many ways of practicing *Chi*, for the purpose of this chapter I invited Taiwanese Grand Master Shiao-Chin Lan, the 1993 and 1997 World Martial Arts Championship Bronze Medal winner of *Tai Chi Chuan*, to demonstrate the practice of *Chi-Kung*

using a very simple approach. This approach consists of two parts: the *Standing Chi-Kung* and the *Sitting Chi-Kung*. For practicing *Standing Chi-Kung*, the exerciser stands with both legs open wide in line with the shoulders and both hands relax beside the body (see Picture 1). Then, keeping breathing controlled, the exerciser slowly inhales and images the *Chi* is directed from *Dan-Tien*, a small spot located 2 inches inside of the navel, to the head with both hands gradually being raised to the chest (see both Picture 2 and 3). Then, continuing to inhale, the hands are lifted to the head (see Picture 4 and 5). Then the exerciser exhales slowly, with both hands down at the two sides of the body, and images the *Chi* directed from the head's *Bai-Hui* (an acupuncture point located in the center of the head) along *Du Mei*, returning to *Dan-Tien* (see Picture 6), then back to the original posture (as in Picture 7) (illustrated and

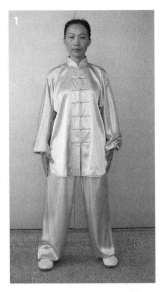
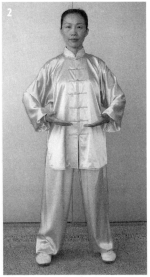
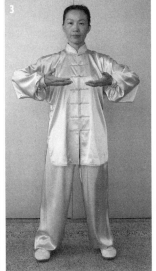
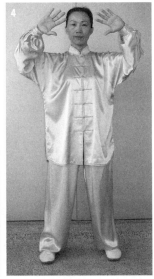

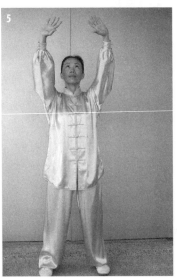
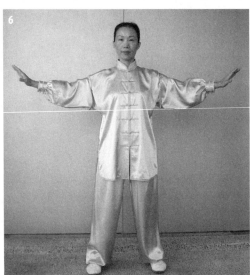
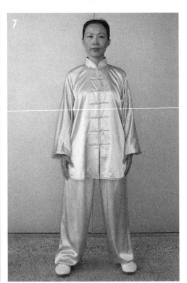

explained by Grand Master Shiao-Chin Lan).

To practice *Sitting Chi-Kung,* which relies heavily on meditation, the exerciser sits cross-legged Yoga-style (see Picture 8). Because the practice of *Sitting Chi-Kung* is totally made up of imagery and meditation, one can not be aware of the overt change of the movements. The exerciser practices *Sitting Chi-Kung* sitting quietly and relaxed, with both eyes slightly closed. When inhaling and exhaling, the exerciser controls the breathing by counting numbers up or down. While inhaling, the exerciser images the *Chi* directed from *Dan-Tien* along *Ren Mei* (i.e., front body central line). And, while exhaling, the exerciser images the *Chi* is directed from the head's *Bai-Hui* back to *Du Mei* (i.e., back body central line). Although making no overt movements, those who practice *Sitting Chi-Kung* concentrate on breathing control by counting numbers upwards, one, two, three, four,

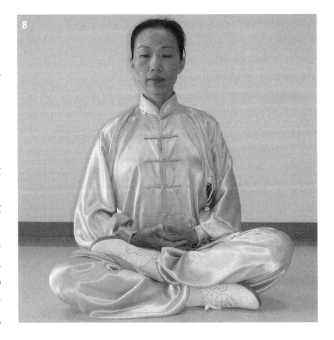

five, etc., depending on one's capacity of the volume of breath. It is recommended that 70% of the capacity to control breath is the most appropriate. That is, when you are maximally able to count from one to ten, counting up to seven is the most appropriate. In addition to counting numbers, imaging the flow of *Chi* is a very important part of *Sitting Chi-Kung*. With a slow and focused mind, those who practice *Sitting Chi-Kung* concentrate on the *Chi* flow along the front line and back line of the body. Then, gradually, imaging *Chi* flow covers the whole body with energy. Or, while inhaling, imaging the *Chi* brings positive powers such as energy, strength, confidence, control, agility, speed, etc., and they will come to you, following the control of *Chi*. On the other hand, while exhaling, imaging *Chi* will take away all the negative powers such as fatigue, tiredness, hatred, anger, confusion, injuries, etc.

There is great deal of evidence of legendary subjective experiences of the benefits of practicing *Chi*, reported by many martial artists as well as fitness instructors. Some of those said that they had experienced an inner-generated greater power (Fogan, 2005; Lam, 2003), reducing stress and anxiety (Burk, 2002; Yu & Hoff, 2000), transmitting of power (Connor, 1992), curing cancer (Yu & Hoff, 2000), and relief of depression (Shirley, 2007). Because the practice of *Chi* has a great deal of similarity to the practice of PST, such as arousal regulation, imagery, attention control, confidence building, and self reinforcement, I will discuss this link in the next part of the chapter.

The Link between *Chi* and Psychological Skills Training

By reading the previous section, readers can gain a better understanding of *Chi,* as well as the relationship between *Chi* and Chinese medicine, the relationship between *Chi* and eastern martial arts, the effects of practicing *Chi*, and how to practice the *Chi*. The following section is intended to underscore the similarities between practicing *Chi* and practicing PST.

Chi and Arousal Regulation

Arousal is used synonymously with the term *activation*, and these terms both refer to the intensity level of behavior (Duffy, 1957). The relationship between arousal and athletic performance is well-documented in sport psychology (e.g., Anshel, 2005; Weinberg & Gould,

2007). To perform their best, athletes must identify the optimal arousal level and learn to regulate it (Landers & Arent, 2001). For methods of identifying the optimal level of arousal, readers can refer to related textbooks (e.g., Nideffer, 1985; Williams & Harris, 2001). As to arousal regulation, Williams and Harris suggested the use of *muscle-to-mind relaxation skills* and/or *mind-to-muscle techniques*.

The practice of *Chi* has advantages over these two approaches. From a *muscle-to-mind* perspective, when practicing *Chi*, martial artists use both breath control and movement control in order to lower undesired high arousal. Such practices lower autonomous nervous system (ANS) functioning because lowered breathing and slow movement slow down the ANS function.

On the other hand, from a *mind-to-muscle* perspective, when practicing *Chi*, exercisers must keep the mind functioning at all times, that is, keep concentrating on breathing control and numbers counting down, and imaging that *Chi* is moving along *Ren-Mei* and *Du-Mei* in order to keep from becoming distracted. At this moment, exercisers must focus their thoughts on the imagery. Therefore, the belief is that *Chi* enables exercisers to become relaxed and focused, which, in turn, makes exercisers perform better in the ensuing sport performance.

As *Chi-Kung* masters state, once exercisers are deeply involved in *Chi*, the exerciser experiences that the mind and body have come together because they take place simultaneously. Sometimes exercisers experience that the mind has imparted to the body, or that the body has imparted to the mind. Furthermore, exercisers will experience with mindfulness that unforced attention accompanies awareness and recognition. These are all the internal experiences of practicing *Chi*. At this moment, because of the mind-body connection, it reduces undesired arousal and leads exercisers to an optimal state.

Chi and Imagery
Imagery is a technique where one creates or recreates an experience in the mind (Weinberg & Gould, 2007). The process of imagery involves recalling experiences (i.e., seeing, tactile, feeling, or hearing) from memory and shaping these experiences into meaningful images. As previously stated, there is an imagery component when practicing *Chi*. Martial artists image the flow of *Chi*, and image how it starts from *Dan-Tien* and flows along two major vessels—*Ren Mei* and *Du Mei. Chi-Kung*

exercisers believe this exercise generates greater power and brings health. Therefore, when practicing *Chi,* exercisers involve many imagery processes, especially guiding the direction of *Chi,* and eventually apply it to single strike such as martial artists' performance.

In his manual *Seven Steps to Peak Performance,* Suinn (1986) introduced a special mental skill to guide one's energy by visualization. He teaches athletes to use visualization in order to image the existence of energy, guide the energy to the tools or equipment that athletes are about to use, or to the space in which they are about to perform, or control the objects coming into one's energy space. The *Chi-Kung* master uses a similar way to transfer power to another person, so as to promote the exerciser's ability (Connor, 1992). Although this is only a legendary tale in martial arts, it is believed that this approach has strong powers of suggestion on those who practice *Chi.* Therefore, although it is the practice of martial arts, it also reflects the characteristics of psychological skills training.

Chi and Confidence Building

Self-confidence is one's belief that he or she can successfully accomplish a required task or desired behavior. Sport psychologists suggest that higher confidence not only arouses positive emotions and facilitates concentration, but also affects goals and performance (Vealey, 1986; Weinberg & Gould, 2007; Zinsser, Bunker, & Williams, 2001). Therefore, how to build and enhance one's confidence is a very important issue in applied sport psychology. Zinsser, Bunker, and Williams (2001) suggested that cognitive strategies, such as thought- and awareness-control and self-talk, are important methods for building athletes' confidence. On the other hand, Weinberg and Gould suggested structuring competition and training conditions so as to allow athletes to gain a feeling of accomplishment and vicarious experience. Using imagery, goal mapping, physical conditioning, and preparation can also improve athletes' confidence. Moreover, Vealey (2001) suggested that strengthening athletes' achievement (mastery and demonstration of ability), self–regulation (physical/mental preparation, physical self-presentation), and social climate (social support, coach's leadership, vicarious experiences, environmental comfort, situational favorableness) all facilitate confidence.

Although these suggestions are very insightful, it remains challenging to determine precisely how an athlete becomes confident before competition. Nideffer (1985) introduced a special technique learned from Aikido that can enhance one's state of confidence during performing, called *centering.* When practicing centering, one has to direct his or her thoughts toward the center of gravity in the body (actually, it is the *Dan-Tien,* where it was previously stated, a small spot located 2 inches inside the navel). Nideffer contended that when the mind rests on this point, one is centered. The feeling of being centered is a strong, confident, anchored kind of feeling.

The practice of *Chi* is similar to centering. When practicing *Chi,* either *Chi-Kung* or *Tai Chi Chuan,* the master will ask exercisers to guide their *Chi* along the *Ren-Mei* and *Du-Mei.* By doing this practice, exercisers concentrate their thoughts on the pathway of *Chi* flow, starting from *Dan-Tien* to *Ren-Mei* and *Du-Mei.* During this imagination, exercisers come to a state of concentration and relaxation, and many sport psychologists suggest that this state is linked to one's confidence (Nideffer, 1985; Vealey, 2001).

Chi and Concentration

Concentration is the key to success and peak performance, as attested by many athletes. For example, Ravizza (1977) interviewed 20 male and female athletes and found that during their peak performance, they experienced total immersion in the activity and a narrow focus of attention. In studies by Garfield and Bennett (1984) and Privette and Bundrick (1997), athletes reported similar experiences, such as extraordinary awareness, a feeling of being completely in control and detached from the external environment and any potential distractions, and focusing fully on the relevant task of the game. To help athletes enhance their concentration during competition, Nideffer (1985) referred to an optimal state of total control called *mind-like-water* by his Aikido master, where the exerciser has to focus on *Ki (Chi).*

Nideffer's (1985) Aikido approach is just like *Chi-Kung.* He taught Tom Petranoff (a former world record javelin thrower) to use centering to control his breath, monitor and relax muscles, and perform visualization during competition. Petranoff's psychological manipulation is very similar to the practice of *Chi-Kung.* To achieve their best performance, many martial artists use *Chi-Kung* to break a stack of bricks, as in Karate, or attack several opponents simultaneously, as in Taekwondo or Aikido, or hit down a wall with bare fists as in Chinese *Kung Fu*. Such performance requires extreme concentration, and Tom and many other great athletes did it.

Chi and Self-Reinforcement

When facing challenges, such as an important competition, the beginning of another training program, or during any occasion in which athletes must affirm themselves, they need self-reinforcement. Generally, reinforcement refers to the use of rewards and punishment that increase or decrease the likelihood of a similar response occurring in the near future (Weinberg & Gould, 2007). Reinforcement is rooted in the theories of behavior modification and operant conditioning by behaviorists such as Skinner (1974). However, there is a way to strengthen one's behavior by internal self-talk such as: "I feel good about myself"; "I am ready for the coming event"; "The training will make me strong and agile"; "I appreciate my teammates' encouragement because I understand that our team will be more cohesive after this session of communication;" etc.

Self-reinforcement is totally self-initiated and directed. Its purpose is to affirm one's decisions and strengthen confidence and determination; particularly, it is helpful for athletes to do this in the moment before competition. Athletes tend to become full of self-doubt and anxiety when competition nears (Hardy, 1996). To avoid unnecessary cognitive anxiety, especially worries and self-doubts, athletes using *Chi* can not only facilitate concentration but also avoid distractions. By controlling breathing such as by counting numbers down or up—along with imagining the power of *Chi*—athletes gain reinforcement before competition, which in turn facilitates better performance.

The Application of *Chi* to Psychological Skills Training

To gain the best results, this chapter recommends following four phases for applying *Chi* in sport settings, including (a) developing the *Chi;* (b) exercising the *Chi;* (c) manipulating the *Chi;* and (d) applying the *Chi*.

Developing the *Chi*

In this stage, athletes need to have an understanding of *Chi* and how it is practiced, and how to learn it during the off-season. I suggest providing athletes with a simple and explicit introduction of what *Chi* is, how it works, and how martial artists use it in their performance. As the way to start, I suggest using breath control and imagination of the *Chi* flow. To practice breath control, the easiest way to do this is to begin at a very small range and move to a wider range of breathing control; for example, inhaling while counting to three and exhaling while counting in reverse from three. Next, athletes can control deeper breathing by inhaling or exhaling to the range of four, to five, to six, and to seven, etc., and practicing deeper and deeper breathing. Also, for maximizing the effect of this practice, the exerciser may concentrate the movement at *Dan-Tien*, that is, the movement of navel inward and outward. As to the imagination of the *Chi* flow, the exerciser can imagine that the *Chi* is moving from *Dan-Tien* along *Ren-Mei* to the head, and then from *Du-Mei* to *Dan-Tien*. These two small practices achieve two major purposes: (a) familiarity with breath control, and (b) experience of the existence of *Chi*. Moreover, to achieve the best development of *Chi*, many martial arts masters suggest exercisers should maintain an appropriate and healthy life style practice, such as diet, physical exercise, daily life schedule, etc. Also, they recommend that maintaining a positive social and spiritual atmosphere, such as harmonious social interaction, positive attitude toward work, promote ethical and moral practices, etc., all contribute to the best development of *Chi*.

Exercising the *Chi*

When athletes are familiar with *Chi* and believe in its existence, they must exercise it. It is best to start with *Standing Chi-Kung* to "see" the flow of *Chi* by slowly raising their hands up to their head, and slowly putting down their hands and exhaling. Further, athletes may use *Sitting Chi-Kung* for meditation and imagination. While sitting alone in a quiet place, such as sitting in front of a desk, athletes may use breathing control and counting down or up to feel and develop the *Chi* and to become familiar with its practice. Athletes may practice *Standing Chi-Kung* and *Sitting Chi-Kung* during their free hours or when they alone. They may practice it before come to training arena, or while they are waiting for the school bus. Like most of PST training 5 to 15 minutes in a single session, and 3 to 5 times per week makes practice perfect. Before learning a new skill or facing an intensive physical conditioning, a short *Chi* practice makes athletes relax and provides concentration to facilitate their performance. Also, when athletes are injured, practicing *Chi* facilitates their rehabilitation and shortens their recovery.

Manipulating the *Chi*

To maximize the effects of *Chi,* athletes need to learn to manipulate it during training and competition. For training, athletes can imagine the flow of *Chi* in sports equipment, clothes, and facilities. To accomplish this, they can imagine the *Chi* is developing in the *Dan-Tien,* through breath control. Then gradually, they can feel the *Chi* flow along *Ren-Mei* and *Du-Mei,* to both hands, and then imagine *Chi* is transferred to the sports equipment, clothes, and facilities. For competition, athletes may stand in front of the competition field, with both eyes focused on the field and imagine that *Chi* is transferred to the field, covering every corner, on the audience, referees, and even the opponents. Also, athletes may imagine that *Chi* controls opponents and eliminates them so to enhance confidence. While performing their skill, athletes may also imagine that *Chi* is gradually transferring to training or competition sites. For example, athletes stare at one location on the field, such as the check point of the high jump, or javelin, or the aiming point of the basketball rim, and imagine that *Chi* has covered these places. At this moment, athletes focus on the chosen spot and make surroundings blurry, and then imagine that *Chi* has covered at these places. Especially, through deeper control and by way of imaging that *Chi* is getting stronger and stronger, athletes feel that they are focused, confident, and ready to perform.

Applying the *Chi*

In this stage, athletes are already mastering the *Chi* so that they can apply it in many occasions. For example, when an important competition is coming, athletes may use *Chi* as a tool to regulate arousal. Before competition, athletes can find a quiet place and use *Sitting Chi-Kung* to allow themselves to become focused and relaxed, so as to achieve a state of optimal confidence and arousal. Or, using *Sitting Chi-Kung* as Nideffer (1985) suggested, they can achieve a state of *"mind-like-water,"* and block out distractions, or feel in control of everything. Sometimes, if necessary, athletes may arrive at the competition site one or two days before competition in order to check the related fields, facilities, or equipment. At this time, they can manipulate *Chi* covering these objects

and gradually bring these objects under their control.

On the other hand, to enhance their confidence, athletes may use *Chi* on sports equipment such as rackets, shoes, clubs, clothes, spikes, and bats, by imaging that *Chi* is being transferred from *Dan-Tien* to these objects. As Suinn (1986) suggested, athletes may focus their sight on these objects and imagine a ray of light covering these objects. When this process is completed, it means that *Chi* is already being transferred, thus helping the athletes to believe these objects are under the covering of their *Chi,* with special magic power, and in turn, building their confidence.

Conclusions

Past research on the psychology of Olympic excellence concluded that world champions and Olympic medalists possessed many exceptional psychological characteristics such as the ability to control and utilize anxiety (Gould, Dieffenbach, & Moffett, 2002; Orlick & Partington, 1988), higher self-confidence and more positive self-talk (Williams & Harris, 2001), and better concentration than unsuccessful Olympians (Orlick & Partington, 1988). However, these exceptional psychological characteristics are believed to be acquired by learning rather than being inherited (Williams & Harris, 2001). Cultivation of athletes with excellent psychological characteristics is a very necessary part of PST for coaches and sport psychologists. The eastern *Chi* concept I introduced in this chapter is an ideal approach to mastering psychological skills. Although there are very few studies in sport psychology examining the effects of *Chi* on athletic performance, evidence from other fields such as medicine and physiology confirm that *Chi* has numerous effects on human physical and immune functioning (e.g., Cicero, 2006; Liu, Li, & Lee, 2007; Wayne et al., 2007).

The approach of *Chi* introduced in this chapter is to synthesize the practice of eastern martial artists, especially from *Chi-Kung,* with a very simple method that allows athletes to learn the fundamental highlights of *Chi*. By practicing *Chi* in four phases, athletes may gain the effects of arousal regulation, imagery, confidence building, concentration, and self-reinforcement, as I discussed in the previous section. Because PST is a systematic and consistent practice of mental or psychological skills for the purpose of enhancing performance, increasing enjoyment, or achieving greater sport and physical activity self-satisfaction (Weinberg & Gould, 2007), I believe that the practice of *Chi* would allow athletes to reduce anxiety, concentrate on the task at hand, enhance confidence, and cope with distractions and adversities, so as to enhance their performance and foster positive sport experiences.

References

Anshel, M. A. (2005). Strategies for preventing and managing stress and anxiety in sport. In D. Hackfort, J. L. Duda, & R. Lidor (Eds.), *Handbook of research in applied sport and exercise psychology: International perspectives* (pp. 199-218). Morgantown, WV: Fitness Information Technology.

Burk, F. (2002). Better breathing reduces stress. *Black Belt, 40,* 30-32.

Choy, P. (1999). *T'ai Chi Chi Kung.* New York: Overlook Press.

Cicero, A. F. G. (2006). Effect of constant Tai Chi practices on blood pressure and heart rate: A 6-month open trial. *British Journal of Sports Medicine, 40,* 888-889.

Connor, D. (1992). *QiGong.* York Beach, ME: Samuel Wiser.

Duffy, E. (1957). The psychological significance of the concept of arousal or activation. *Psychological Review, 64,* 265-275.

Dunn, T. (1990). *T'ai Chi ruler.* Berkeley, CA: North Atlantic Books.

Fogan, S. (2005). The ultimate weapon. *Black Belt, 43,* 96-99.

Garfield, C. A., & Bennett, H. Z. (1984). *Peak performance: Mental training techniques of the world's greatest athletes.* Los Angeles: Tarcher.

Gould, D., Dieffenbach, K., & Moffett, A. (2002). Psychological characteristics and their development in Olympic champions. *Journal of Applied Sport Psychology, 14,* 172-204.

Hardy, L. (1996). Testing the predictions of the cusp catastrophe model of anxiety and performance. *The Sport Psychologist, 10,* 140-156.

Huang, W. S. (1984). *Fundamentals of Tai Chi Ch'uan.* Hong Kong: South Sky Book.

Lam, K. C. (2003). *Chi Kung: Way of power.* Champaign, IL: Human Kinetics.

Landers, D. M., & Arent, S. M. (2001). Physical activity and metal health. In R. Singer, H. Hausenblas, & C. Janelle (Eds.), *Handbook of sport psychology* (2nd ed., pp. 740-765). New York: Wiley.

Liu, J., Li, B., & Lee, A. (2007). The effects of Tai Chi training on improving physical functions in patients with coronary heart diseases. *Research Quarterly for Exercise and Sport, 78,* 32.

Nideffer, R. M. (1985). *Athletes' guide to mental training.* Champaign, IL: Human Kinetics.

Orlick, T., & Partington, J. (1988). Mental links to excellence. *The Sport Psychologist, 2,* 105-130.

Privette, G., & Bundrick, C. M. (1997). Psychological processes of peak, average, and failing performance in sport. *International Journal of Sport Psychology, 28,* 323-334.

Ravizza, K. (1977). Peak experiences in sport. *Journal of Humanistic Psychology, 17,* 35-40.

Shirley, A. (2007). Qigong relieves depression in older adults. *IDEA Fitness Journal, 41,* 99.

Skinner, B. F. (1974). *About behaviorism.* New York: Knopf.

Suinn, R. M. (1986). *Seven steps to peak performance.* Toronto: Hans Huber Publishers.

Sun, W. Y., & Li, X. J. (1997). *Chi-Kung.* New York: Sterling Publishing.

Vealey, R. S. (1986). Conceptualization of sport-confidence and competitive orientation: Preliminary investigation and instrument development. *Journal of Sport Psychology, 8,* 221-246.

Vealey, R. (2001). Understanding and enhancing self-confidence in athletes. In R. Singer, H. Hausenblas, & C. Janelle (Eds.), *Handbook of sport psychology* (2nd ed., pp. 550-565). New York: Wiley.

Wayne, P., Kiel, D., Krebs, D., Davis, R., Savetsky-German, J., Connelly, M., et al. (2007). The effects of Tai Chi on bone mineral density in postmenopausal women: A systematic review. *Archives of Physical Medicine and Rehabilitation, 88,* 673-680.

Weinberg, R. S., & Gould, D. (2007). *Foundations of sport and exercise psychology* (4th ed.). Champaign, IL: Human Kinetics.

Williams, J., & Harris, D. V. (2001). Relaxation and energizing techniques for regulation of arousal. In J. Williams (Ed.), *Applied sport psychology: Personal growth to peak performance* (pp. 229-246). Mountain View, CA: Mayfield.

Yang, J. M. (1990). *Chi Kung: Health and martial arts.* Boston: YMAA Publication Center.

Yu, W. M., & Hoff, T. M. (2000). *QiGong : The power to cure cancer.* Inside Kung-Fu, November, 91-95.

Zinsser, N., Bunker, L., & Williams, J. (2001). Cognitive techniques for building confidence and enhancing performance. In J. Williams (Ed.), *Applied sport psychology: Personal growth to peak performance* (pp. 284-311). Mountain View, CA: Mayfield.

Index

About the Editors

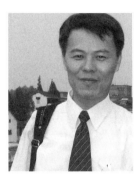

Tsung-Min Hung

Dr. Tsung-Min Hung is a professor in the Department of Physical Education at the National Taiwan Normal University (Taiwan), with an area of expertise in psychophysiology of sport and exercise. He has been the sport psychology consultant for Taiwan's elite athletes for the past 10 years. Dr. Hung's research interests include the psychophysiological signature of optimal motor performance and psychophysiological consequences of physical activity. He has published more than 40 articles in peer-reviewed journals and made more than 80 presentations at international conferences. Dr. Hung is currently serving as president of the Society for Sport and Exercise Psychology of Taiwan (2008-2009). He is also a committee member for both the International Society of Sport Psychology and the Society for Psychophysiological Research.

Ronnie Lidor

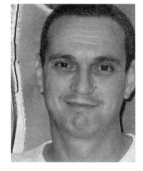

Dr. Ronnie Lidor is an associate professor at the Zinman College of Physical Education and Sport Sciences at the Wingate Institute, and is on the Faculty of Education at the University of Haifa (Israel). His main areas of research are cognitive strategies, talent detection, and early development in sport. Dr. Lidor has published more than 90 articles, book chapters, and proceedings chapters, in English and in Hebrew. His articles have been published in many respected journals such as *The Sport Psychologist, Human Performance, Journal of Sports Sciences, International Journal of Sport Psychology, International Journal of Sport and Exercise Psychology, Psychology of Sport and Exercise, Journal of Aging and Physical Activity, Pediatric Exercise Science,* and *Physical Education and Sport Pedagogy.* He is the co-editor of several books, among them *Sport Psychology: Linking Theory and Practice* (1999), *The Psychology of Team Sports* (2003), and *Handbook of Research in Applied Sport and Exercise Psychology: International Perspectives* (2005), all published by Fitness Information Technology (USA). From 1997 to 2001 Dr. Lidor served as president of the Israeli Society for Sport Psychology and Sociology. Since 1997, he has been a member of the Managing Council of the International Society of Sport Psychology (ISSP). In 2001, he was elected as the secretary general of ISSP. He has been the editor of *Movement – Journal of Physical Education and Sport Sciences* (Hebrew) since 1999.

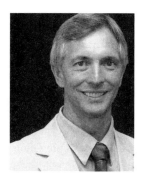

Dieter Hackfort

Dr. Dieter Hackfort is a professor of sport and exercise psychology, and is currently serving as dean of ASPIRE Academy for Sports Excellence in Doha, Qatar. He received his doctoral degree in 1983 from the German Sports University. In 1986, he was a visiting professor at the Center for Behavioral Medicine and Health Psychology at the University of South Florida in Tampa, and received tenure at the University of Heidelberg. In 1991, he was the founding professor for the Institute of Sport Science at the University AF Munich. Since 1986, he has served as a counselor for professional performers and athletes of various sports at the Olympic Centers in Germany. Dr. Hackfort's research has been published in 25 books and edited volumes, and in more than 150 contributions to national and international journals. In 1984, he received an award from the German Sports Federation for the best research in the social sciences 1983-1984 (Carl-Diem-Plaque), and in 2001 he received the Honour Award of the International Society of Sport Psychology (ISSP) in recognition of his significant contributions to national and international sport psychology through leadership, research, and personal service. In 1999, he was appointed Honour Professor of Wuhan Institute of Physical Education, China. He is currently the president of the ISSP.

About the Authors

Abderrahim "Abdou" Baria

Dr. Abderrahim "Abdou" Baria is a professor of sport psychology and the head of the Department of Physical Education at the Ecole Normale Supérieure in Casablanca, Morocco. Dr. Baria holds a master's degree from the University of Montréal (1987) and a PhD from the University of Ottawa, Canada (1994), both supervised by John H. Salmela. Dr. Baria is currently the president of the Moroccan Association of Sport Psychology and a member of the Managing Council of the International Society of Sport Psychology. He is also involved with Moroccan professional golfers as a performance consultant. His research interests focus on cross-cultural studies in sport psychology, sport excellence, and coach expertise development. He has had papers published in refereed international and national journals (in French and in English) and has made presentations at international and national congresses and seminars. He served as an assistant editor for the *International Journal of Sport Psychology* from 1991 to 1995, and has provided peer review services to research journals in French and English.

Jean Côté

Dr. Jean Côté is a professor and director of the School of Kinesiology and Health Studies at Queen's University at Kingston (Canada). His research interests are in the areas of children in sport, sport expertise, positive youth development, and coaching. Dr. Côté is, or has been, on the editorial boards of the *Journal of Applied Sport Psychology, The Sport Psychologist, Revue International des Sciences du Sport et de l'Education Physique,* and *Physical Education and Sport Pedagogy*. He is currently co-editor of the *International Journal of Sport and Exercise Psychology*. Dr. Côté holds cross appointments as a visiting professor at the Carnegie Research Institute, Leeds Metropolitan in the UK, and the School of Human Movement Studies at the University of Queensland in Australia.

Dong-Yang Fong

Dr. Dong-Yang Fong is a professor of sport and exercise psychology at National Taipei University of Technology (Taiwan), where he is the director of the Laboratory of Sport Science. Dr. Fong's research interests include mental training, peak performance, anxiety, and psychophysiology. With the financial support of the National Science Council, he has explored the effect of Qikong on mental health and has developed a training program for aging adults. From 2003 to 2006 he served as a sport psychology consultant for the Olympic and Asian Games athletes. He is a fellow of the Society for Sport and Exercise Psychology of Taiwan.

Liu Hao

Liu Hao is currently a doctoral student and is working with Dr. Dieter Hackfort at ASPIRE Academy for Sports Excellence in Doha, Qatar. He earned his bachelor's and master's degrees in sport science at Wuhan Institute of Physical Education, China. After that, he worked at Hong Kong Sports Institute as a research assistant. He has been involved in several research projects related to achievement motivation, stress management, and self-concept, as well as mental skills training for junior athletes. His current focus is on the development of special training programs in the framework of the Mental Test and Training System (MTTS).

Keith Henschen

Dr. Keith Henschen is a professor in the Department of Exercise and Sport Science at the University of Utah, with an area of expertise in applied sport psychology. He has published more than 200 articles, 35 book chapters, five monographs, co-authored five books, and has made more than 400 presentations. He has served as president (1997-1998) of the American Alliance of Health, Physical Education, Recreation and Dance, and also served as president (2001-2005) of the International Society of Sport Psychology. He has consulted with numerous Olympic, professional, and world class performers. He has been the sport psychology consultant for the Utah Jazz professional basketball team for the past 20 years.

Conor Kilgallen

Conor Kilgallen is currently working as a sport psychology officer at ASPIRE Academy for Sports Excellence in Doha, Qatar. There, his main focus is on applied work, particularly with ASPIRE's soccer players. Before joining ASPIRE in 2006, he worked for *Sport Psychology Ireland*, where he consulted extensively with both elite and amateur sports people in a wide variety of sports.

Po-Yi Lin

Po-I Lin, MS, graduated from the Taipei Physical Education College with a major in sport psychophysiology. He was a lecturer of physical education in college. He is currently preparing for language qualification to apply for a doctoral program in the United States. His research interests include biofeedback training and concentration enhancement issues, physical activity, and cognitive performance. His master's thesis found that heart rate biofeedback training can effectively regulate heart rate deceleration and enhance archery performance.

Li-Chuan Lo

Li-Chuan Lo is a doctoral student and currently working with Dr. Bradley Hatfield in the Department of Kinesiology at the University of Maryland. Her research interests are in the area of sport psychology and cognitive motor neuroscience. Specifically, she is interested in the emotional impact on brain dynamics and precision motor performance, utilizing psychophysiological methods in her research. She earned her BS in physical education and MS in exercise and sport science in Taiwan, and has had several years of working experience with children in elementary school.

Frank J. H. Lu

Dr. Frank J. H. Lu is a professor at the Graduate Institute of Physical Education, the National Taiwan Sport University. He completed his doctoral degree in 1998 at the University of North Carolina at Greensboro. He was the president of the Society for Sport and Exercise Psychology of Taiwan from 2005 to 2007, and an active member in international sport psychology bodies, such as the Association of Applied Sport Psychology, International Society of Sport Psychology, and Asian South Pacific Association of Sport Psychology. His major research interest is the social and psychological aspects of youth sport issues, such as burnout, fear of failure, and social support. Regarding applied practices, he combines Western psychological skills training and

Eastern martial arts concepts of *Chi* to enhance Taiwanese athletes' performance and personal growth.

Dimitrios Milosis

Dr. Dimitrios Milosis holds a diploma in physical education and sport science (Aristotle University of Thessaloniki, Greece), a diploma in business administration (University of Macedonia, Thessaloniki, Greece), an MSc in teaching in physical education (Aristotle University of Thessaloniki, Greece), and a PhD in psychology of education (Democritus University of Thrace, Greece). He has been a gymnastics coach since 1990 and has taught physical education in schools since 1995. During the past three years he has supervised the practicum of the physical education student teachers in the Aristotle University of Thessaloniki. He co-authored two books for public education in Greece, as well as more than 20 articles and book chapters in international and Greek journals and congress proceedings in the areas of interdisciplinary teaching, self-regulation, motivational climate, and goal orientations in physical education.

Athanasios Papaioannou

Dr. Athanasios Papaioannou has a diploma in physical education and sport science from the Aristotle University of Thessaloniki, Greece. He has an MPhil degree in the psychology of physical activity, and a PhD in education and psychology from the University of Manchester, UK. From 1994 until 2005 he was affiliated with the Democritus University of Thrace, Greece. He is currently a professor at the University of Thessaly, Greece, and director of a master's program in sport and exercise psychology. He teaches courses in sport and exercise psychology, psychology for physical educators, statistics, and research methods. He has more than 50 international publications in the area of motivation in physical activity and sport, and he has co-authored five books in Greece in the area of psychology for physical educators and coaches. He is co-editor of the *International Journal of Sport & Exercise Psychology* and is an editorial board member of *Psychology of Sport and Exercise*. Dr. Papaioannou was the director of the 10th World Congress of Sport Psychology and he is currently the treasurer of the International Society of Sport Psychology.

Al Petitpas

Dr. Al Petitpas is a professor in the Psychology Department at Springfield College, where he directs the Center for Youth Development and Research. He is a licensed psychologist in Massachusetts, a Fellow in Division 47 of the American Psychological Association, and a certified consultant of the Association for the Applied Sport Psychology. He has provided consulting services to a wide range of sport organizations, including Play It Smart, The First Tee, Montreal Alouettes, NCAA, NBA, NFL, U.S. Olympic Committee, U.S. Ski Team, and the LPGA.

Rico Schuijers

Dr. Rico Schuijers is a sport psychologist. He studied sport psychology in Nijmegen, the Netherlands, and started his own consulting company in 1990. In addition to working as a sport psychologist in the Netherlands, Dr. Schuijers worked on his doctoral thesis from 1996 to 2003 at the Sporthochschule of Köln in Germany, where he received his doctoral degree in 2003. He is the chairman of the Society for Sport Psychology in the Netherlands and a member of the Managing Council of the International Society on Sport Psychology. His daily work consists of training and coaching elite athletes. He works with multiple national teams and individual athletes in different sports, focusing mainly on the Olympics. He also works for the air force and with Dutch air traffic controllers of Schiphol Airport and European air traffic controllers of Eurocontrol in Maastricht, the Netherlands. Topics of his work are: performing under pressure; stress management; coping with change; awareness of individual differences; team-building; challenging/motivating athletes in performing at their best; and concentration and self-confidence. He has published two books in Dutch.

Sidonio Serpa

Dr. Sidonio Serpa studied physical education and psychology in Lisbon, Portugal, and earned his PhD in sport sciences from the Technical University of Lisbon, where he is a professor of sport psychology and chair of the unit. His main research areas are coach-athlete relationships, psychology of doping, and psychology of sport excellence and talent. He coordinates the sport psychology services of the Centre of Sport Excellence of Lisbon, and has worked as a consultant for many top-level athletes and medalists in European, World, and Olympic competitions in several sports. He served as a sport psychologist in the Olympic Games of Atlanta and Sydney, and was included in the staff of the Portuguese sailing team. Dr. Serpa is currently vice president of the International Society of Sport Psychology and is a member of the European "Forum of Applied Sport Psychologists in Topsport."

Natalia Stambulova

Dr. Natalia Stambulova is a professor in sport and exercise psychology in the School of Social and Health Sciences at Halmstad University, Sweden. Her professional experiences in sport psychology reflect her three decades of work as a teacher, researcher, and consultant in the USSR/Russia and, since 2001, in Sweden. Her athletic background is in figure skating on the level of the USSR national team. She received her first PhD (1978) in developmental psychology at the Leningrad State University, and the second (1999) in sport psychology at the St. Petersburg State University of Physical Education and Sport. Her research and publications relate mainly to the topic of athletic career, with an emphasis on career transitions and crises. In applied work, her specializations are helping athletes in crisis, and consulting with athletes and coaches on various athletic/life career issues. She has been a member of the Managing Council of the International Society of Sport Psychology since 2001. In 2004, she received the Distinguished International Scholar Award of the Association of Applied Sport Psychology.

Traci Statler

Dr. Traci Statler is an assistant professor in the Department of Kinesiology at California State Fullerton, with an expertise in the area of applied sport and performance psychology. Her primary research interests include the "art" of excellence in performance, the psychology of high-level disabled sport performance, and the psychology of injury and rehabilitation, with numerous professional presentations in these areas. She has been working in the area of applied sport psychology for the last 15 years and currently serves as a performance psychology consultant to USA Track & Field and to a variety of collegiate athletic programs, as well as conducting individual performance enhancement sessions with professional athletes, police officers, and fire fighters in southern California. Dr. Statler has also served as a member of the Managing Council of the International Society of Sport Psychology for the last four years.

Judy L. Van Raalte

Dr. Judy L. Van Raalte is a professor of psychology at Springfield College in Springfield, MA, where she is the co-director of the Athletic Counseling master's program. She has worked with elite and professional athletes in the United States and around the world. Dr. Van Raalte's research interests include body issues, professional issues in sport psychology, self-talk, and sport injury. With the financial support of the National Institutes of Mental Health, she has developed and evaluated the effectiveness of a multimedia CD-ROM for college student eating disorder education. She has also published more than 70 articles in peer-reviewed journals, presented at conferences in 11 countries, written four books, and served as an executive producer of 15 sport psychology videos. She is a certified consultant (Association for the Advancement of Applied Sport Psychology) and is listed on the United States Olympic Committee Sport Psychology Registry. From 2003 to 2004, she served as president of the American Psychological Association's Division of Exercise and Sport Psychology (Division 47), and from 2005 to 2009 as the vice president of the International Society of Sport Psychology. Dr. Van Raalte is a fellow of both the American Psychological Association and the Association for Applied Sport Psychology.

Yung-Shun Wang

Yung-Shun Wang, MS, graduated from the Taipei Physical Education College with a major in sport psychophysiology. He has established a sport-related mental skill training office that helps athletes improve their mental skills, mainly via neurofeedback training. His research focus is on neurofeedback training and sport performance enhancement issues.